CW00494354

COLOUR GUIDE

# Orthodontics and Paediatric Dentistry

Declan Millett BDSc, DDS, FDS(RCPSGlasg), DOrthRCSEng, MOrthRCSEng
Senior Lecturer in Orthodontics
University of Glasgow Dental School
Honorary Consultant in Orthodontics
Glasgow Dental Hospital and School
North Glasgow University Hospitals NHS Trust
Glasgow

Richard Welbury MB BS, BDS, PhD, FDSRCS
Consultant in Paediatric Dentistry
Newcastle upon Tyne Dental Hospital
Newcastle upon Tyne Hospitals NHS Trust
Honorary Senior Clinical Lecturer
University of Newcastle upon Tyne
Newcastle upon Tyne

CHURCHILL LIVINGSTONE

EDINBURGH LONDON NEW YORK PHILADELPHIA ST LOUIS SYDNEY TORONTO 2000

CHURCHILL LIVINGSTONE
An imprint of Harcourt Publishers Limited

© Harcourt Publishers Limited 2000

is a registered trademark of Harcourt Publishers Limited

The right of Declan Millett and Richard Welbury to be identified as authors of this work has been asserted by them in accordance with the Copyright, Designs and Patents Act 1988

All rights reserved. No part of this publication may be reproduced, stored in a retrieval system, or transmitted in any form or by any means, electronic, mechanical, photocopying, recording or otherwise, without either the prior permission of the publishers (Harcourt Publishers Limited, Harcourt Place, 32 Jamestown Road, London NW1 7BY), or a licence permitting restricted copying in the United Kingdom issued by the Copyright Licensing Agency, 90 Tottenham Court Road, London W1P 0LP.

ISBN 0443 06287 0

**British Library Cataloguing in Publication Data**
A catalogue record for this book is available from the British Library.

**Library of Congress Cataloging in Publication Data**
A catalog record for this book is available from the Library of Congress.

**Note**
Medical knowledge is constantly changing. As new information becomes available, changes in treatment, procedures, equipment and the use of drugs become necessary. The authors and the publishers have, as far as it is possible, taken care to ensure that the information given in this text is accurate and up to date. However, readers are strongly advised to confirm that the information, especially with regard to drug usage, complies with the latest legislation and standards of practice.

Printed in China
SWTC/01

The publisher's policy is to use **paper manufactured from sustainable forests**

*For Churchill Livingstone*

*Commissioning Editor:*
Mike Parkinson
*Project Development Manager:*
Sarah Keer-Keer & Siân Jarman
*Project Controller:* Frances Affleck
*Designer:* Erik Bigland

# Preface

The clinical interface of orthodontics and paediatric dentistry is broad. Increasingly, for the undergraduate, teaching and examinations in these specialties are combined to promote a holistic approach to dental care for the child and adolescent patient. This concise colour guide aims, therefore, to cover major clinical aspects of orthodontic and paediatric dental practice in a format suitable for quick reference and revision purposes. It assumes a good working knowledge and competence in history taking/clinical examination as well as an understanding of the principles of treatment planning for both disciplines. Space restrictions preclude the inclusion of some topics which are dealt with comprehensively in specialist texts (listed under Recommended Reading). Although directed primarily at the undergraduate, we hope that this colour guide will be of value also to the junior postgraduate and to those preparing for membership examinations.

We wish to acknowledge particularly the help and support of Mrs K. Shepherd, Mrs G. Drake, Mr J. Davies (Glasgow Dental Hospital and School) and Mr B. Hill and Mrs J. Howarth (Newcastle upon Tyne Dental Hospital) in the preparation of photographic material. We would also like to thank Mr A. Shaw (Fig. 27b), Miss D. Fung (Fig. 28), Mr J. G. McLennan (Figs. 68, 100, 101, 103), Dr L-H. Teh (Figs. 78, 84) and Miss J. Hickman (Fig. 85). The Index of Orthodontic Treatment Need is reproduced by kind permission of VUMAN Limited. We also thank the staff of Harcourt Health Sciences who have been very helpful throughout. Finally we pay special tribute to Eithne Johnstone for her considerable skill and advice in preparing and text editing the initial drafts of the manuscript.

Glasgow and Newcastle upon Tyne — D. T. M.
2000 — R. R. W.

# Contents

# 1 / Normal development of the dentition and occlusion

## Normal development

*Definition*

The changes one would expect in the 'average' child. For average eruption dates see page 83.

## Primary dentition

Incisors are usually spaced and upright. No spacing indicates the probable crowding of successors (Fig. 1). 'Primate' spacing may exist distal to $\underline{c}$s and mesial to $\bar{c}$s. Distal surfaces of es are flush in most cases. By 5–6 years, an edge-to-edge occlusion with incisor attrition is common.

## Primary to mixed dentition

- $\overline{1|1}$ or $\overline{6}$s are usually the first to erupt; mild incisor crowding is common (Fig. 2) but tends to resolve by 9 years with an increase of about 2–3 mm in intercanine width.
- Space for $\underline{21|12}$ is provided by existing incisor spacing, by intercanine width growth, and by their greater proclination than $\underline{ba|ab}$.
- $\underline{1|1}$ are usually distally inclined initially; median diastema reduces with $\underline{2|2}$ eruption. As $\underline{3|3}$ migrate and press on the roots of $\underline{2|2}$, their crowns, and to a lesser extent those of $\underline{1|1}$, are frequently flared distally with a median diastema – 'ugly duckling' stage (Fig. 3). This usually corrects as $\underline{3}$s erupt.
- Space for 3, 4, 5s is provided by the slightly greater mesiodistal width of c, d, es. Greater leeway space in the mandible (~2–2.5 mm) than in the maxilla (~1–1.5 mm) with mandibular growth creates a Class I molar relationship.

## Dental arch development

With the exception of intercanine width increase, dental arch size alters minimally after the primary dentition erupts. Permanent molars are accommodated by growth at the back of the arch. Alveolar bone growth maintains occlusal contact as the face grows vertically.

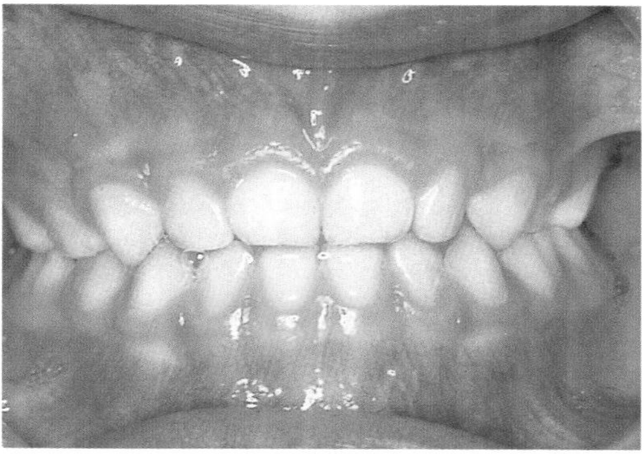

**Fig. 1** Unspaced primary dentition.

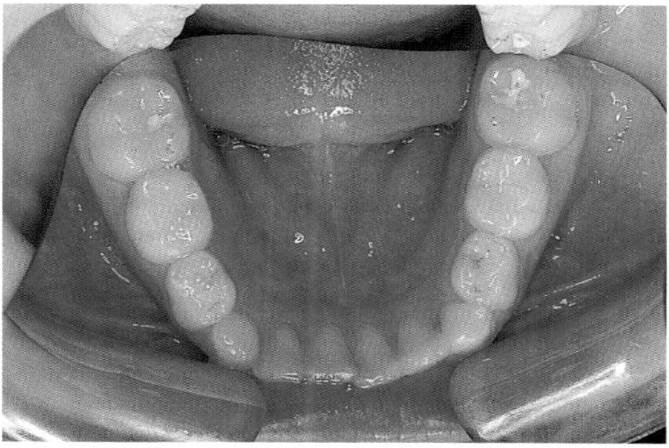

**Fig. 2** Mild incisor crowding (aged 8).

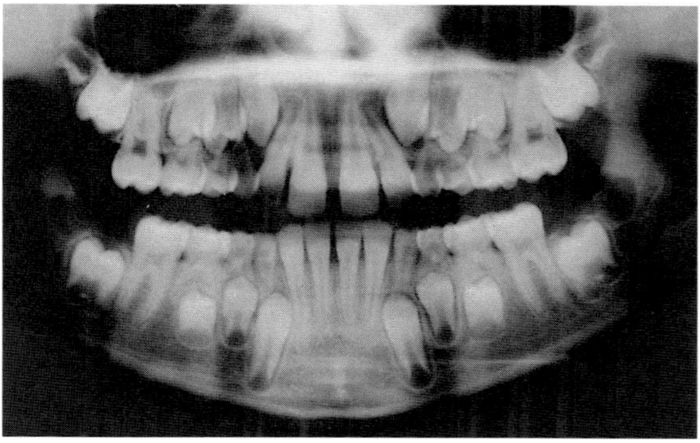

**Fig. 3** 'Ugly duckling' stage.

# Normal permanent occlusion

## Static occlusal relations (Andrews' six keys)

- *Molar relationship* (Fig. 4). Distal surface of the distal marginal ridge of $\underline{6}$ contacts and occludes with the mesial surface of the mesial marginal ridge of $\overline{7}$; the mesiobuccal cusp of $\underline{6}$ lies in the groove between the mesial and middle cusps of $\overline{6}$; the mesiolingual cusp of $\underline{6}$ seats in the central fossa of $\overline{6}$.
- *Crown angulation.* Gingival aspect of the long axis of each crown lies distal to its occlusal aspect.
- *Crown inclination.* The gingival aspect of the labial surface of the crown of $\underline{21|12}$ lies palatal to the incisal aspect. Otherwise, the gingival aspect of the labial or buccal surface of the crowns of all other teeth lies labial or buccal to the incisal/occlusal aspect.
- No rotations.
- No spaces.
- Flat or mildly increased ($\leq$1.5 mm) curve of Spee.

## Functional occlusal relations

- Centric relation should coincide with centric occlusion.
- A working side canine rise (Fig. 5) or group function should be present on lateral excursions, with no occlusal contact on the non-working side; the incisors should only contact in protrusion.

## Maturational changes in the occlusion

- Increase in lower incisor crowding (Fig. 6).
- Slight increase in interincisal angle with incisor uprighting.
- Slight increase in mandibular prognathism.

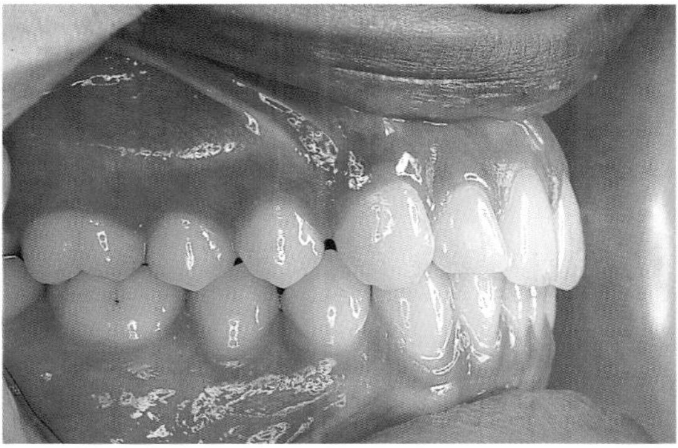

**Fig. 4** Normal molar relationship.

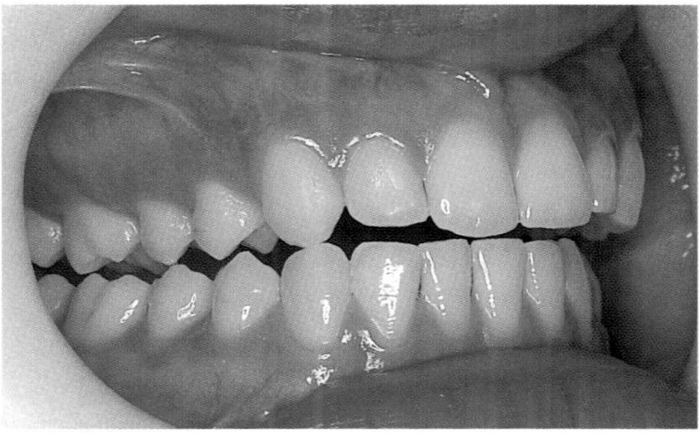

**Fig. 5** Canine guided right lateral excursion; note that no non-working side contacts were present.

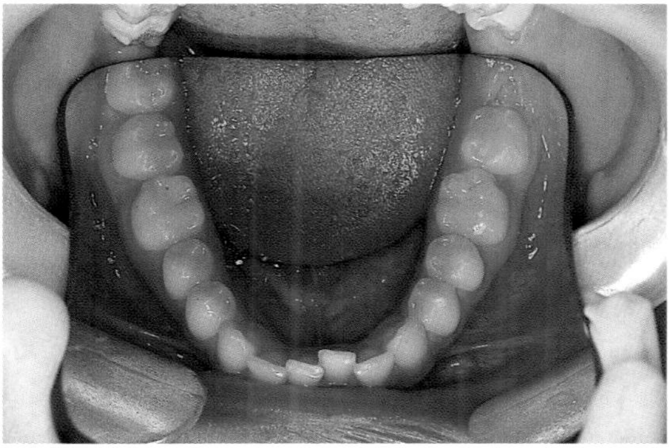

**Fig. 6** Late lower incisor crowding.

# 2 / Malocclusion

*Definition* An unacceptable deviation – aesthetically and/or functionally – from the 'ideal' occlusion.

*Prevalence* Varies with age, racial origin and assessment method.

## Classification for diagnostic purposes

### Angle's classification based on molar relationship

*Class I (normal or neutrocclusion).* Mesiobuccal cusp of $\underline{6}$ occludes in the buccal groove of $\overline{6}$ (Fig. 7). Discrepancies of ≤ half a cusp width were also regarded as Class I by Angle.

*Class II (postnormal occlusion or distocclusion).* Mesiobuccal cusp of $\underline{6}$ occludes anterior to the buccal groove of $\overline{6}$ (Figs 8, 9).

*Class III (prenormal occlusion or mesiocclusion).* Mesiobuccal cusp of $\underline{6}$ occludes posterior to the buccal groove of $\overline{6}$ (Fig. 10).

### British Standards Institute classification based on incisor relationship

*Class I.* Lower incisor edges occlude with or lie immediately below the cingulum plateau (middle third of the palatal surface) of the upper incisors (Fig. 7).

*Class II Division 1.* Class II: lower incisor edges lie posterior to the cingulum plateau of the upper incisors. Division 1: there is an increase in overjet and the upper incisors are proclined or of average inclination (Fig. 8).

*Class II Division 2.* Class II as above. Division 2: upper central incisors are retroclined; overjet is usually minimal but may be increased (Fig. 9).

*Class III.* Lower incisor edges lie anterior to the cingulum plateau of the upper incisors; overjet is reduced or reversed (Fig. 10).

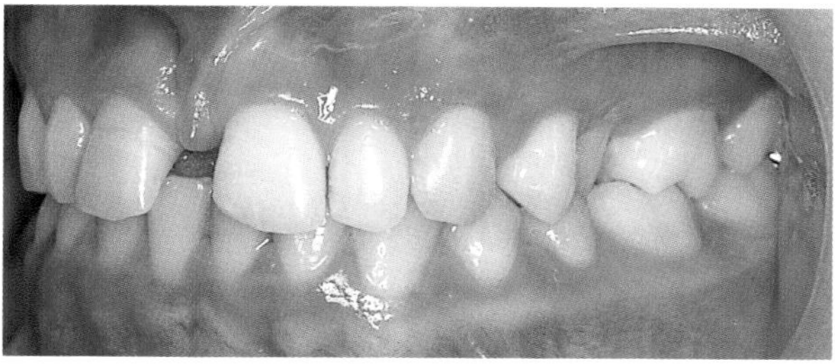

**Fig. 7** Class I molar and incisor relationships.

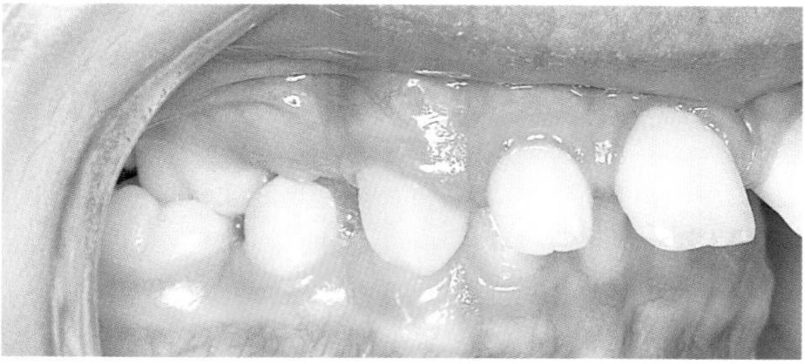

**Fig. 8** Class II molar/II Division 1 incisor relationship.

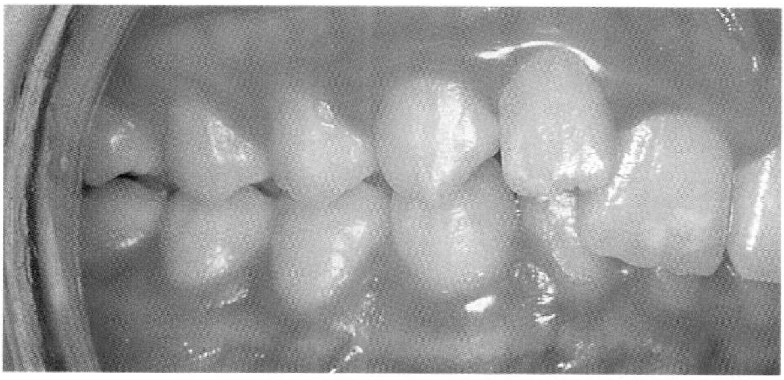

**Fig. 9** Half unit Class II molar/II Division 2 incisor relationship.

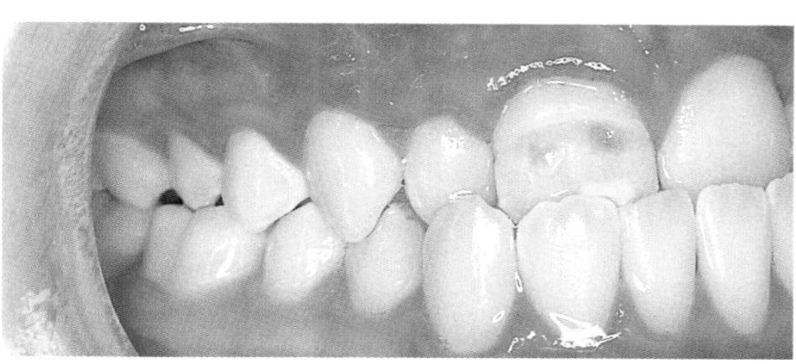

**Fig. 10** Class III molar and incisor relationships.

## Classification to assess treatment need

*Index of orthodontic treatment need (IOTN)*

Helps to identify those malocclusions most likely to benefit in dental health and appearance from orthodontic treatment; comprises two components:
- Dental health component (DHC)
- Aesthetic component (AC).

*Dental health component (DHC)* (Fig. 11a). Malocclusion categorised objectively into five treatment grades, from no need (Grade 1) to very great need (Grade 5). Occlusal features are assessed in the following order: missing teeth (M), overjet (O), crossbite (C), displacement of contact points, i.e. crowding (D), overbite (O), giving the acronym MOCDO. A ruler (Fig. 11b) facilitates the grading process.

| GRADE 5 (Need treatment) | |
|---|---|
| 5.i | Impeded eruption of teeth (except for third molars) due to crowding, displacement, the presence of supernumerary teeth, retained deciduous teeth and any pathological cause. |
| 5.h | Extensive hypodontia with restorative implications (more than 1 tooth missing in any quadrant) requiring pre-restorative orthodontics. |
| 5.a | Increased overjet greater than 9mm. |
| 5.m | Reverse overjet greater than 3.5mm with reported masticatory and speech difficulties. |
| 5.p | Defects of cleft lip and palate and other craniofacial anomalies. |
| 5.s | Submerged deciduous teeth. |

| GRADE 4 (Need treatment) | |
|---|---|
| 4.h | Less extensive hypodontia requiring prerestorative orthodontics or orthodontic space closure to obviate the need for a prosthesis. |
| 4.a | Increased overjet greater than 6mm but less than or equal to 9mm. |
| 4.b | Reverse overjet greater than 3.5mm with no masticatory or speech difficulties. |
| 4.m | Reverse overjet greater than 1mm but less than 3.5mm with recorded masticatory and speech difficulties. |
| 4.c | Anterior or posterior crossbites with greater than 2mm discrepancy between retruded contact position and intercuspal position. |
| 4.1 | Posterior lingual crossbite with no functional occlusal contact in one or both buccal segments. |
| 4.d | Severe contact point displacements greater than 4mm. |
| 4.e | Extreme lateral or anterior open bites greater than 4mm. |
| 4.f | Increased and complete overbite with gingival or palatal trauma. |
| 4.t | Partially erupted teeth, tipped and impacted against adjacent teeth. |
| 4.x | Presence of supernumerary teeth. |

| GRADE 3 (Borderline need) | |
|---|---|
| 3.a | Increased overjet greater than 3.5mm but less than or equal to 6mm. with incompetent lips. |
| 3.b | Reverse overjet greater than 1mm but less than or equal to 3.5mm. |
| 3.c | Anterior or posterior crossbites with greater than 1mm but less than or equal to 2mm discrepancy between retruded contact position and intercuspal position. |
| 3.d | Contact point displacements greater than 2mm but less than or equal to 4mm. |
| 3.e | Lateral or anterior open bite greater than 2mm but less than or equal to 4mm. |
| 3.f | Deep overbite complete on gingival or palatal tissues but no trauma. |

| GRADE 2 (Little) | |
|---|---|
| 2.a | Increased overjet greater than 3.5mm but less than or equal to 6mm with competent lips. |
| 2.b | Reverse overjet greater than 0mm but less than or equal to 1mm. |
| 2.c | Anterior or posterior crossbite with less than or equal to 1mm discrepancy between retruded contact position and intercuspal position. |
| 2.d | Contact point displacements greater than 1mm but less than or equal to 2mm. |
| 2.e | Anterior or posterior openbite greater than 1mm but less than or equal to 2mm |
| 2.f | Increased overbite greater than or equal to 3.5mm without gingival contact. |
| 2.g | Pre-normal or post-normal occlusions with no other anomalies (includes up to half a unit discrepancy). |

| GRADE 1 (None) | |
|---|---|
| 1. | Extremely minor malocclusions including contact point displacements less than 1mm. |

**Fig. 11a** Dental health component of the index of orthodontic treatment need.

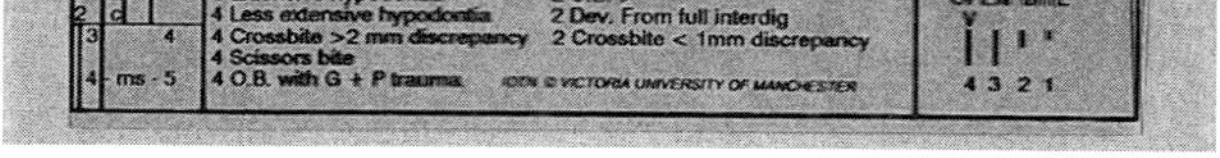


**Fig. 11b** Index of orthodontic treatment need ruler.

*Index of orthodontic treatment need (IOTN) (contd)*

*Aesthetic component (AC)* (Fig. 12). Uses a set of 10 photographs of anterior occlusion with increasing aesthetic impairment. Assessment is made by selecting the photograph thought to match the aesthetic handicap of the case. Treatment need is categorised as follows: score 1–2 = no need; 3–7 = borderline need; 8–10 = definite need. The method suffers from subjectivity.

## Classification to assess treatment outcome

Objective assessment using DHC of IOTN, and subjective assessment by AC of IOTN. Peer assessment rating (PAR) may be recorded also. Six aspects, each given a different weighting, of the pre- and post-treatment occlusion may be assessed from study models with the aid of a ruler (Fig. 13). The percentage change in the PAR score measures success. A 70% reduction in the PAR score indicates 'greatly improved' occlusion, while 'worse/no different' is indicated by ≤ 20% reduction in score.

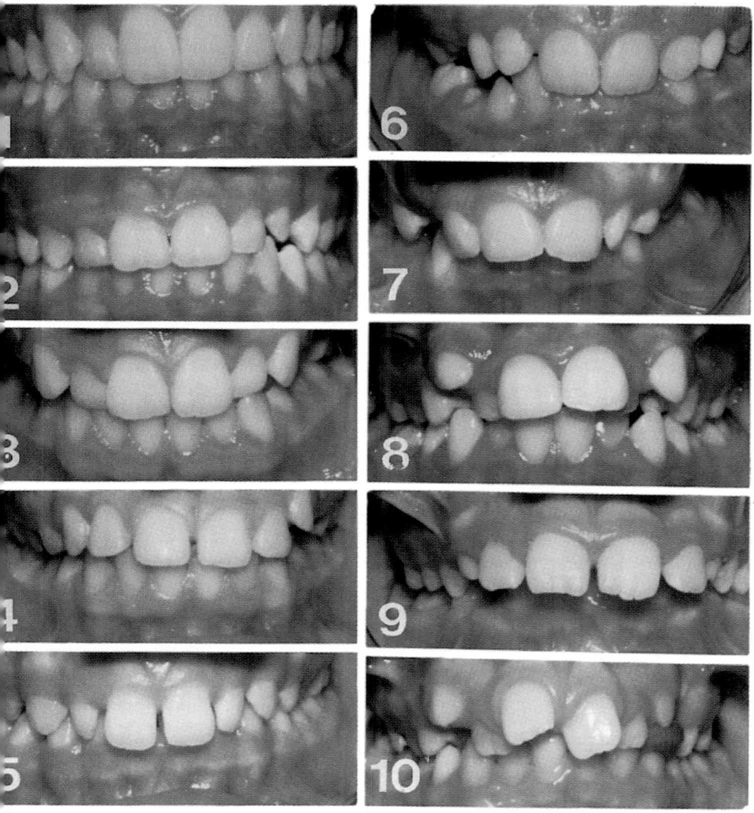


**Fig. 12** Aesthetic component of the index of orthodontic treatment need.

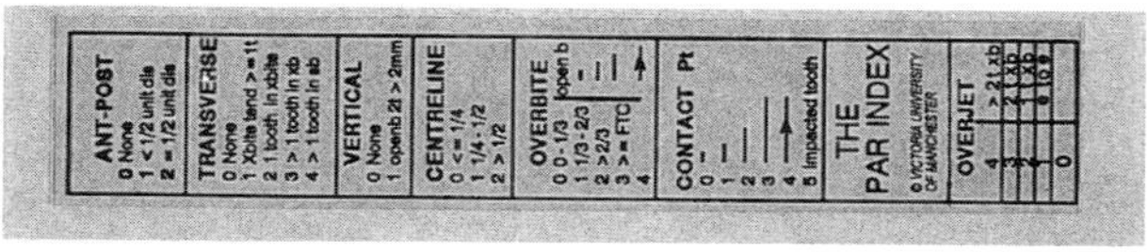


**Fig. 13** Peer assessment rating ruler.

# 3 / Cephalometric analysis

*Definition*

Evaluation and interpretation of both lateral and posteroanterior (PA) radiographs of the head (usually confined to the former).

*Taking the radiograph*

Standardised technique to ensure reproducibility and minimise magnification:

Frankfort plane horizontal, ear posts in the external auditory canal with the central X-ray beam directed through them, teeth in centric occlusion, X-ray source at a fixed distance to the midsagittal plane (about 152.5 cm) and to the film (see Fig. 14). Collimate the beam to reduce radiation exposure. An aluminium wedge enables the soft tissues to be demonstrated (Fig. 15).

*Indications*

When anteroposterior and/or vertical skeletal discrepancies are present (Fig. 15); when anteroposterior incisor movement is planned in these cases.

*Uses of lateral cephalometric analysis*

- To aid diagnosis by allowing dental and skeletal characteristics of a malocclusion to be assessed.
- To check treatment progress during fixed or functional treatments and to monitor the position of unerupted teeth.
- To assess treatment and growth changes by superimposing radiographs or tracings on reasonably stable areas: cranial base or its approximation (S–N line holding at S; Fig. 16); anterior vault of the palate; Bjork's structures in the mandible.

## Aim and objective of cephalometric analysis

*Aim*

To assess the anteroposterior and vertical relationships of the upper and lower teeth with supporting alveolar bone to their respective maxillary and mandibular bases and to the cranial base.

*Objective*

To compare the patient to normal population standards appropriate for his/her racial group, identifying any differences between the two.

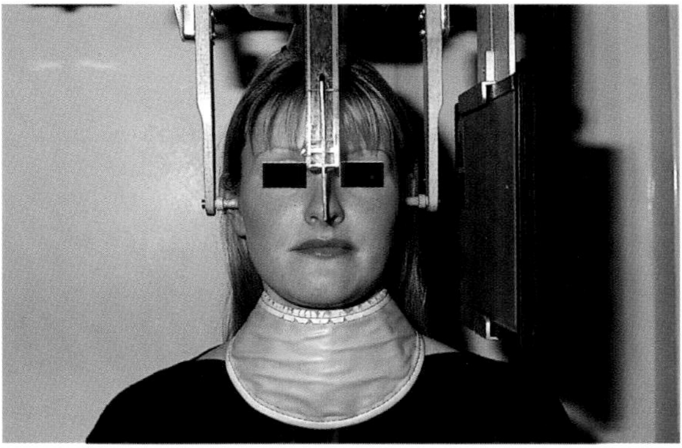

**Fig. 14** Patient in a cephalostat.

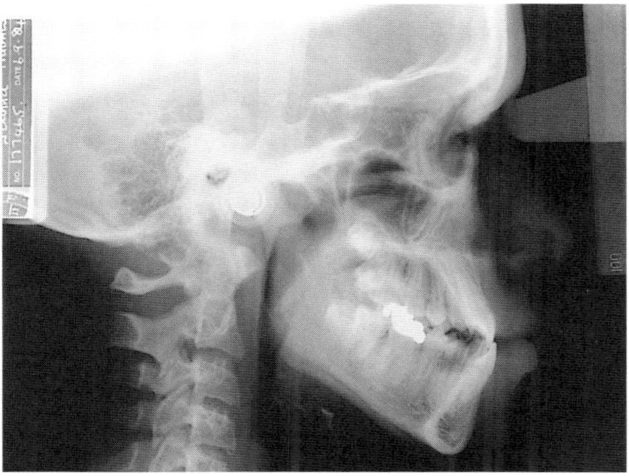

**Fig. 15** Lateral cephalometric radiograph.

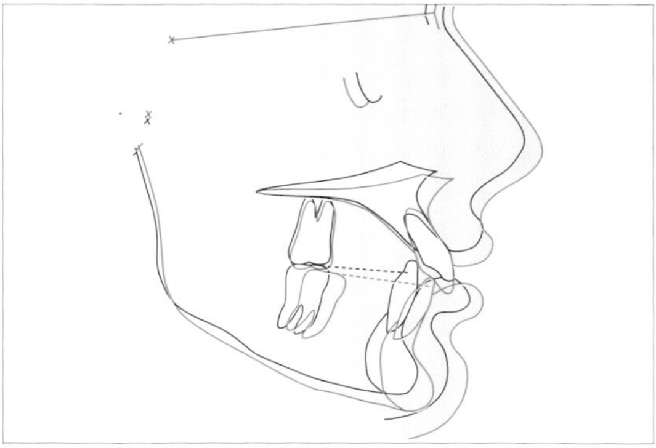

**Fig. 16** Superimposed computer-generated tracings on S–N at S (black = pre-treatment; red = post-treatment).

## Practice of cephalometric analysis

Ensure that teeth are in occlusion and that the patient is not postured forward.

In a darkened room, by tracing or digitising, calculate angular/linear measurements; identify the points and planes shown in Fig. 17; always trace the most prominent image. For structures with two images (e.g. the mandibular border), trace both and take the average for gonion.

## Cephalometric interpretation

For Caucasians, compare individual values with Eastman norms:
SNA 81° ± 3°; SNB 78° ± 3°; ANB 3° ± 2°; S–N/Max plane 8° ± 3°; $\underline{1}$ to Max plane 109° ± 6°; $\overline{1}$ to Mand plane 93° ± 6°; Interincisal angle 135° ± 10°; MMPA 27° ± 4°; Facial % 55 ± 2%.

*Skeletal relationships*

*A–P.* If SNA < or > 81° and S–N/Max PL within 8° ± 3°, correct ANB as follows: for every °SNA > 81°, subtract 0.5° from ANB value and vice versa.

*Vertical.* MMPA and Facial % should lend support to each other usually.

*Tooth position*

- To assess if overjet reduction is possible by tipping movement, do a prognosis tracing (Fig. 18), or for every 1 mm of overjet reduction subtract 2.5° from $\underline{1}$ inclination. If the final inclination is not < 95° to maxillary plane, tipping is acceptable.
- Check $\overline{1}$ angulation to mandibular plane in conjunction with ANB and MMPA. There is an inverse relationship between $\overline{1}$ angulation and MMPA.
- Interincisal angle: as this increases, overbite deepens.
- $\overline{1}$ to APo: this is an aesthetic reference line but it is unwise to use for treatment planning purposes.

*Soft tissue analysis*

Useful for orthognathic planning.
- *Holdaway line*: lower lip should be ±1 mm to this line.
- *Ricketts' E-line*: lower lip should be 2 mm (±2 mm) in front of this with the upper lip slightly behind.

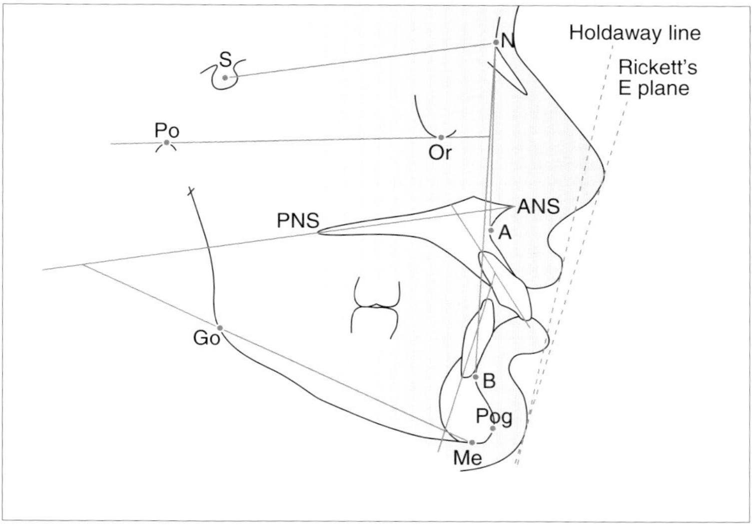


**Fig. 17** Cephalometric points, planes and angles. Points: S (Sella); N (Nasion); Po (Porion); Or (Orbitale); A ('A'point); B ('B'point); Pog (Pogonion); Me (Menton); Go (Gonion). Planes: Frankfort (Po–Or); Maxillary (ANS–PNS); Mandibular (Go–Me).

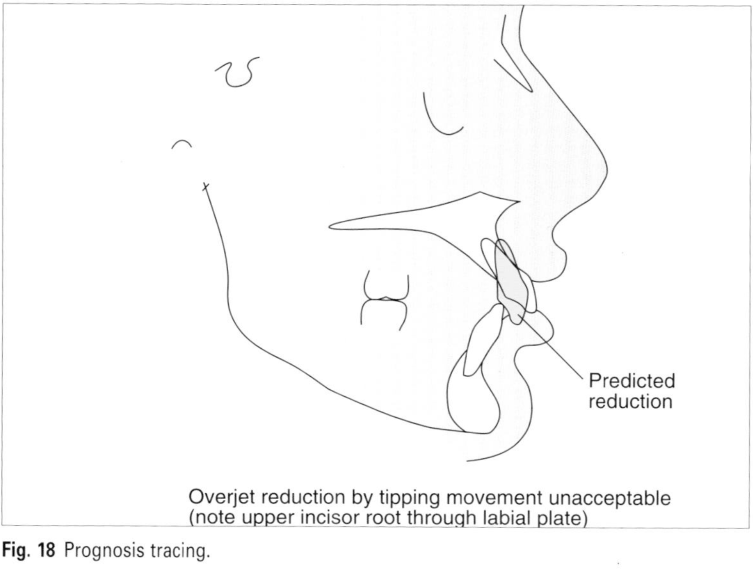


**Fig. 18** Prognosis tracing.

# 4 / Mixed dentition I

## Early loss of primary teeth

*Causes*

Caries (Fig. 19), premature exfoliation often in severely crowded cases (Fig. 20), or planned to encourage mesial drift of the buccal segments.

*Factors determining the outcome*

Patient's age, degree of crowding, tooth extracted, arch from which it is removed, type of occlusion – all these factors influence the potential for crowding to be concentrated at the extraction site. The effects of the early loss of each tooth are:

*Loss of a or b.* Tends to have minimal effect as it usually exfoliates in the early mixed dentition; if the loss is due to trauma, this may lead to dilaceration of its successor.

*Loss of c.* Unilateral loss leads to centreline shift (Fig. 20); balance extraction to prevent this.

*Loss of d.* Occasionally centreline shift follows (Fig. 19); assess the need for balancing extraction by checking midlines at reviews.

*Loss of e.* First permanent molar migrates mesially and may lead to considerable space loss if extraction is carried out before the permanent molar erupts (Fig. 21). In very crowded cases, loss of e before age 7 may promote centreline shift – consider balancing or compensating extractions.

*To minimise undesirable sequelae*

Always consider balancing (extraction of a tooth on the opposite side of the arch which may not be the same tooth type) or compensating (extraction of the equivalent opposing tooth) for any extraction.

Consider space maintenance when premature loss of a tooth will promote crowding in an otherwise acceptable occlusion, or in severely crowded cases where space from later mid-arch extraction of permanent teeth will just be sufficient for alignment of the remaining units. Use upper removable appliance or lingual arch.

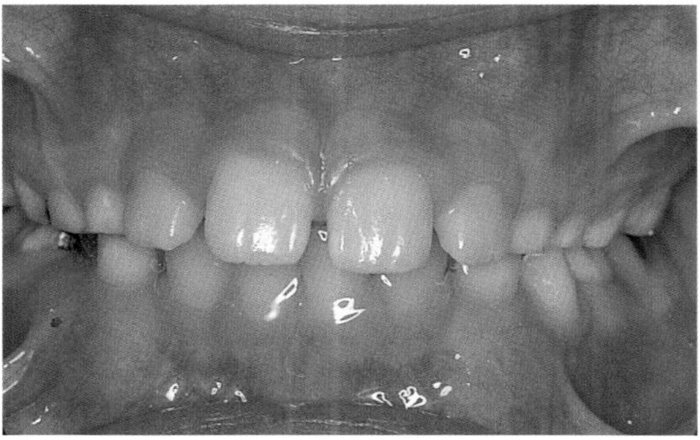

**Fig. 19** Early loss of $\overline{d|}$ due to caries; centreline shift.

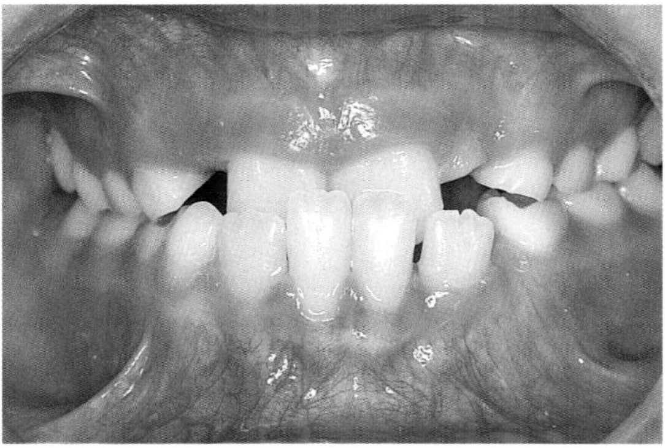

**Fig. 20** Early loss of $\overline{|c}$ due to marked crowding; centreline shift.

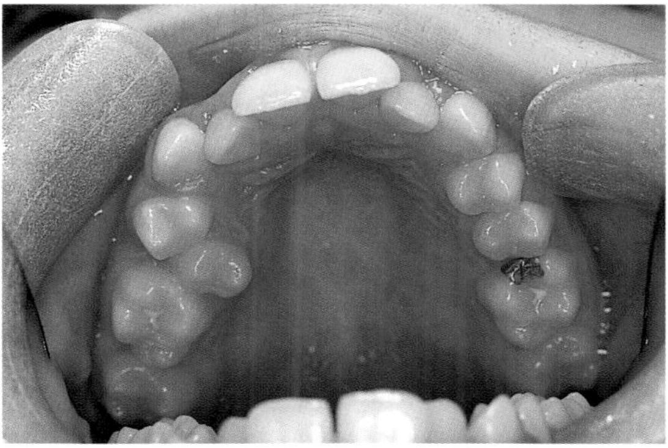

**Fig. 21** Severe crowding due to early loss of $\underline{e|}$.

# Serial extraction

*Definition*

Ascribed by Kjellgren* in 1948 to the following:
- Extraction of cs at age 8.5–9.5 years to encourage the alignment of permanent incisors.
- Extraction of ds about 1 year later to encourage the eruption of 4s.
- Extraction of 4s as 3s are erupting.

*Intention*

To remove the need for appliance therapy.

*Indications*

Works best in Class I cases at about 9 years with moderate crowding, average overbite and a full complement of teeth, where there is no doubt about the long-term prognosis of 6s.

*Shortcomings*

- Seldom removes need for further appliance therapy.
- As three episodes of extractions are required, often under general anaesthesia, the full extent of the original technique is never adopted nowadays.

*Contemporary view*

Consider removal of $\underline{c}$s:
- when $\underline{2}$ erupting in potential crossbite (Fig. 22a)
- to create space for proclination of $\underline{2}$ or the eruption of an incisor when a supernumerary has delayed its appearance
- to promote alignment of a palatally displaced $\underline{3}$ (Fig. 23).

Consider removal of $\overline{c}$s:
- to facilitate lingual movement of a lower incisor with reduced periodontal support
- to allow lingual movement of the lower labial segment in some Class III cases (Fig. 22a, b).

* Kjellgren B 1948 Serial extraction as a corrective procedure in dental orthopaedic therapy. Acta Odontologica Scandinavica 8: 17–43

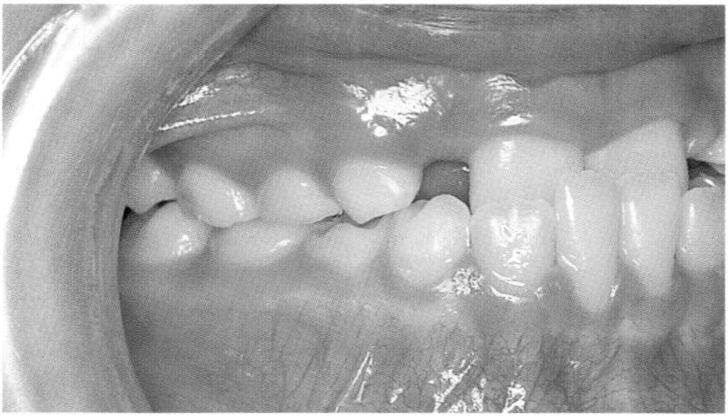

**Fig. 22a** Crossbite 1|1; potential crossbite 2|2; periodontal trauma 1|1.

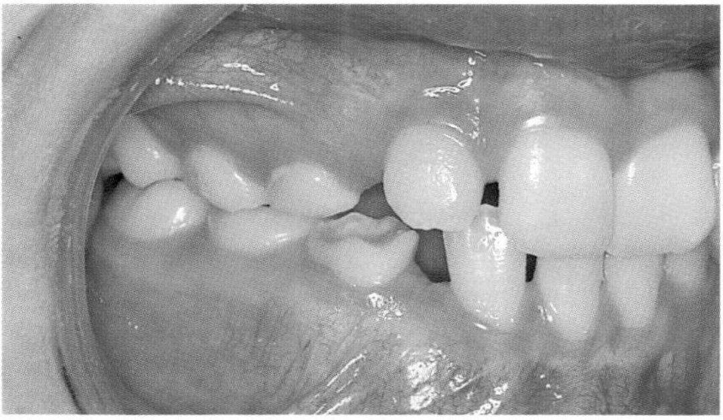

**Fig. 22b** Following extraction of cs and proclination of 1|1.

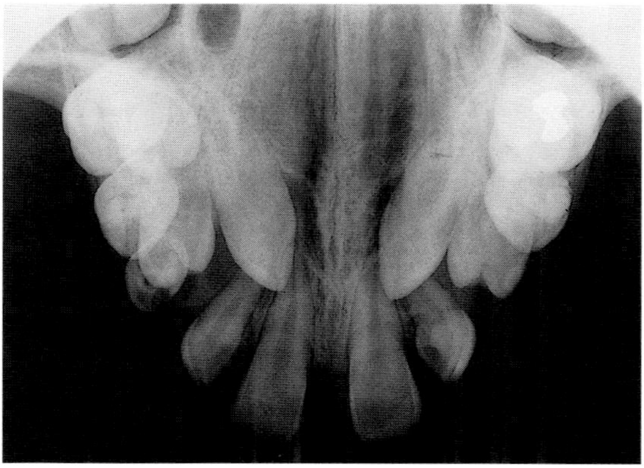

**Fig. 23** 3|3 palatal; position confirmed with DPT (see Fig. 42); cs removed to encourage the alignment of 3s.

*Orthodontic management*

## Supernumerary teeth (see also p. 101)

### Mesiodens

*Conical.* These commonly exist between 1|1 (Fig. 24), often singularly, but sometimes in combination with others of similar form.

*Treatment*:

a. None – if it/they are well above the apices of 1|1, and if there is no risk of damage to adjacent teeth with tooth movement, leave and observe
b. Remove – if it/they are displacing adjacent teeth producing a large diastema or delaying eruption of 1. Also remove a conical supernumerary if it erupts.

*Tuberculate.* The most common cause of unerupted 1 (Fig. 25). May be barrel-shaped.

*Treatment*: remove supernumerary and any retained primary incisors followed by bonding of gold chain or a magnet to the unerupted incisor to allow provision for alignment if spontaneous eruption is not forthcoming within 18 months of surgery. Often removal of cs is also required and URA to move 2|2 distally to create space for 1.

*Supplemental.* Resembles a normal tooth in morphology and commonly produces crowding or displacement of teeth (Fig. 26).

*Treatment*: extract the tooth most dissimilar to the contralateral tooth, provided the more normal tooth is not severely displaced.

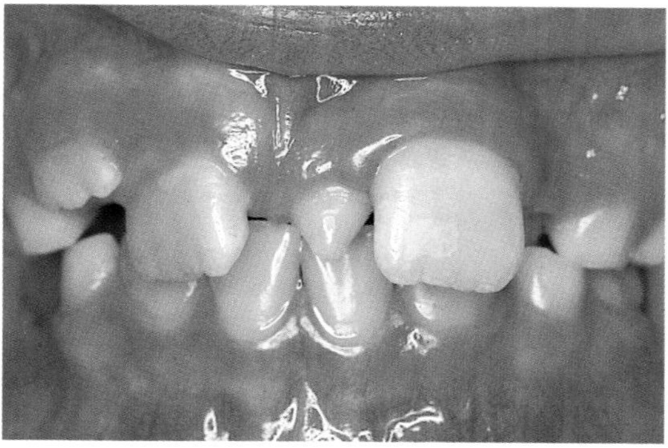

**Fig. 24** Erupted conical mesiodens.

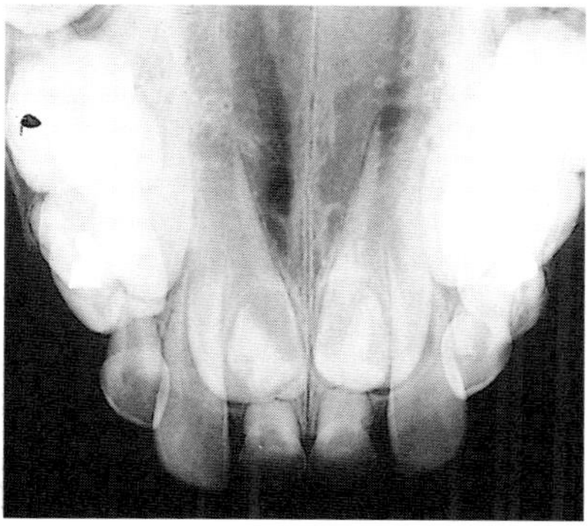

**Fig. 25** Unerupted 1|1 due to two tuberculate mesiodens.

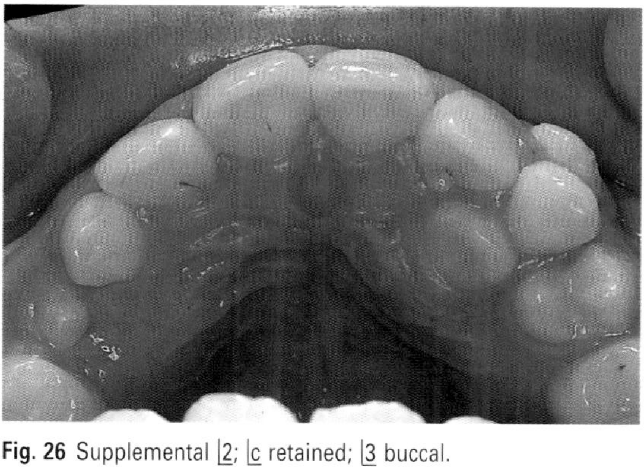

**Fig. 26** Supplemental |2; |c retained; |3 buccal.

# Hypodontia (see also pp. 23, 101)

*Orthodontic management*

*Third molars.* Avoid extraction of 7 for distal movement; calcification of 8 commences at 8–14 years of age.

*Upper lateral incisors.* (Fig. 27a) Options are to open, to maintain or to close the space. The decision depends on: the patient's attitude to treatment; anteroposterior and vertical skeletal relationships; colour, size, shape and inclination of canine and incisor teeth; whether arches are spaced or crowded; the occlusion of the buccal segments. Carry out a diagnostic set-up on duplicate study models with joint consultation with a restorative colleague.

Extract $\underline{c}$s early in crowded cases to facilitate mesial drift of posterior teeth; use a fixed appliance to align and approximate $\underline{31|13}$ followed by bonded retention and recontouring of $\underline{3}$s. If the decision is made to maintain or open the space, it may be filled by autotransplantation of a lower premolar (where this is being removed for relief of crowding), or by the provision of a partial denture or resin bonded bridge (Fig. 27b), or by an implant.

*Second premolars.* Retain e if the arch is uncrowded and place occlusal onlay if it starts to submerge. Remove e after 2s erupt if there is mild crowding, to encourage space closure, but leave and remove later if the crowding is severe. (NB: watch for late developing $\overline{5}$.)

*Lower incisors.* A fixed appliance is required to close the space in a crowded arch or to open space in an uncrowded arch prior to prosthetic replacement of $\overline{1|1}$.

*If there is severe hypodontia.* (Fig. 28) Multidisciplinary care is needed.

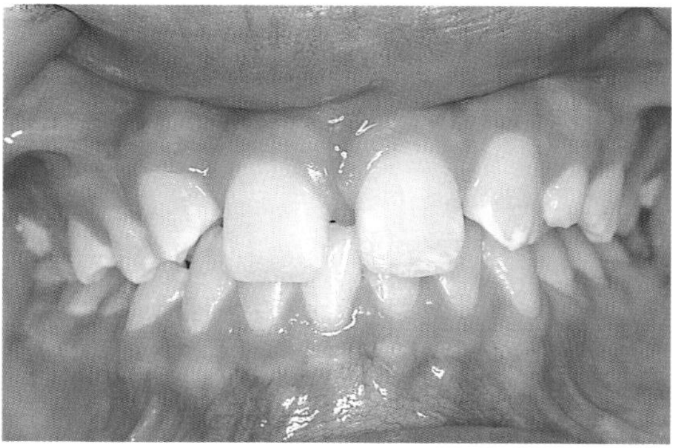

**Fig. 27a** Absent 2|2.

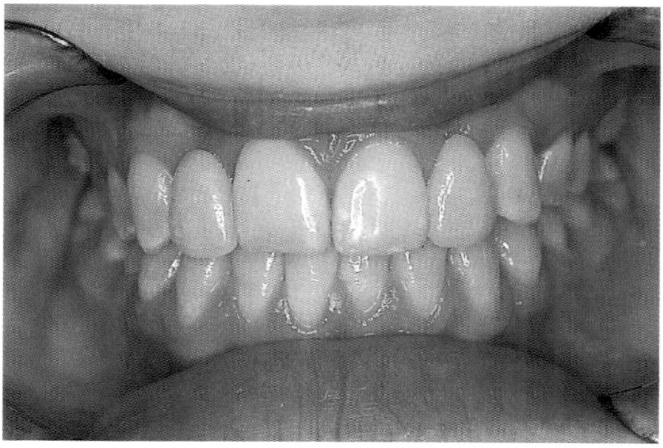

**Fg. 27b** After appliance therapy; resin retained bridges for 2s.

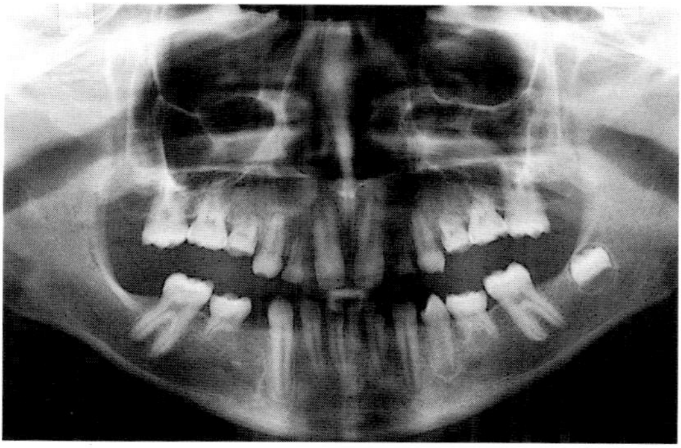

**Fig. 28** Severe hypodontia.

# 6 / Mixed dentition III

## Buccal segment problems

### Retained primary tooth

*Aetiology* — Absent (Fig. 29) or ectopic position of successor.

*Management*

- *If successor is absent*: assess crowding in the quadrant and consider removal.
- *If successor is unerupted and ectopic*: consider removal to encourage alignment if mildly ectopic; otherwise it may be better to accept.
- *If successor is erupting*: remove the primary tooth if it is deflecting the eruption path.

### Infra-occluded primary molars

*Prevalence* — 8–14%.

*Aetiology* — Ankylosis of a tooth while alveolar growth and eruption of the adjacent teeth continues (Fig. 30).

*Management*

- *Keep under observation*: if a permanent successor is present as exfoliation is likely at a similar time to the opposite number in the same arch.
- *Remove*: if a permanent successor is absent or if submergence extends below the gingival level, or if root formation on permanent successor is complete (see also p. 21).

### Impacted $\underline{6}$ (Fig. 30)

*Prevalence* — 2–6% (20–25% in cleft lip with/without palate).

*Aetiology* — Crowding; large crown of $\underline{6}$; eruption path of $\underline{6}$ is too mesial.

*Management*

*Observe.* May correct spontaneously but this is rare after 8 years.

*Active treatment.* Brass wire separators in mild cases. Use appliance to move $\underline{6}$ distally in more severe cases. Also consider the loss of $\underline{e}$ if there is symptomatic resorption with pulpal involvement, or to facilitate restoration of $\underline{6}$. Manage the resulting crowding later.

### Posterior crossbite with mandibular displacement (Fig. 31)

*Aetiology* — Often follows prolonged digit or thumb-sucking.

*Management* — Grind cs may lead to correction; arch expansion with URA and midline screw or quadhelix (see p. 53).

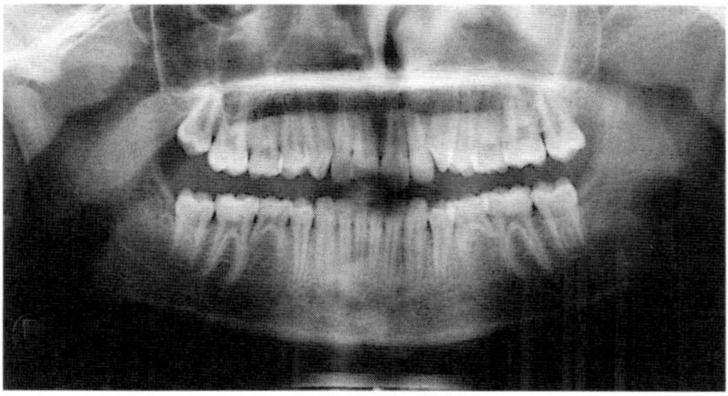

**Fig. 29** Retained es with absent 5s.

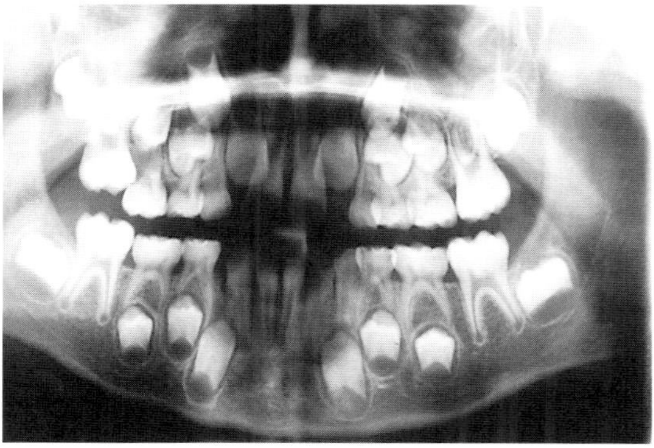

**Fig. 30** Infra-occluded $\overline{ed|de}$; impacted $\underline{6|}$.

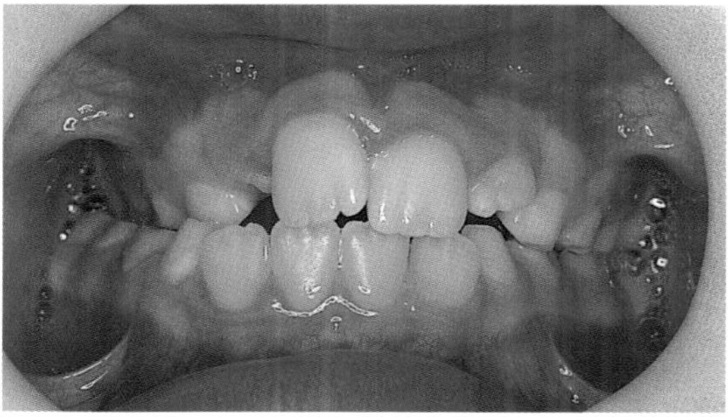

**Fig. 31** Right posterior crossbite with associated displacement.

**First permanent molars (FPM) with poor long-term prognosis**

*Aetiology*

Caries (Fig. 32) or enamel hypoplasia.

*Management*

Timely removal of poor quality FPM may lead to spontaneous correction of malocclusion in certain cases (Figs 33 & 34) but does little to relieve incisor crowding or to correct an incisor relationship unless appliance therapy is instituted. A 'cook-book' approach to each case with poor quality FPM is not possible. Some guidelines, however, are given below:

- Institute preventive measures.
- Assess the patient's motivation for orthodontic treatment and level of dental awareness.
- Ensure that all permanent teeth, particularly 5s, 8s, present radiographically and all others are of good prognosis.
- Avoid extraction of FPM in a quadrant with an absent tooth, or in uncrowded arches.
- Consider balancing or compensating for extraction of a FPM (Figs 33 & 34).
- Timing of extraction of $\overline{6}$: this is best when the bifurcation of $\overline{7}$s is calcifying (Fig. 33) aged approximately 8.5–9.5 years, and moderate premolar crowding is present.
- The timing of the extraction of $\underline{6}$ is less important due to its distal tilt and downward and forward eruption path.
- Extraction of $\underline{6}$ is best delayed
  - — in Class III cases until the incisor crossbite is corrected
  - — in Class II Division 1 cases until $\underline{7}$s erupt
  - — in severely crowded cases until $\underline{7}$s erupt.
- Extraction of $\overline{6}$ may be deferred until $\overline{7}$s erupt in Class III cases with marked incisor crowding.
- Monitor the eruption of 7s and 8s.

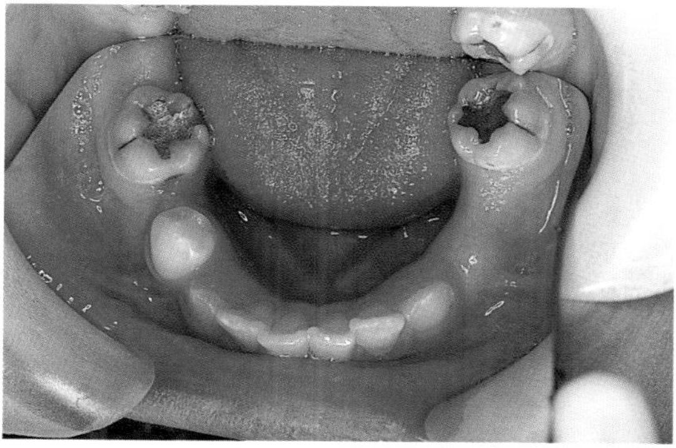

**Fig. 32** Restored and carious first permanent molars.

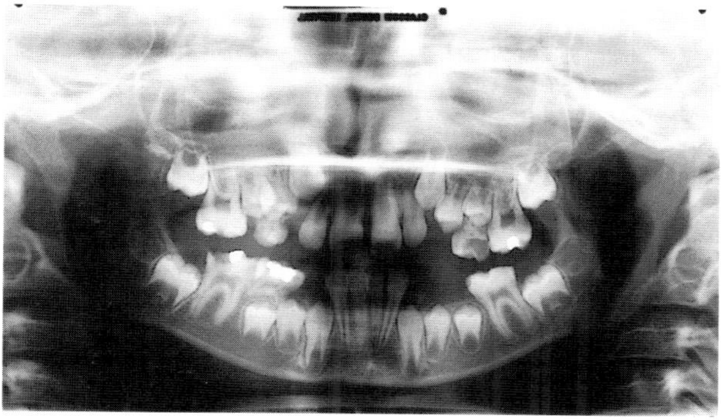

**Fig. 33** Hypoplastic, restored and carious first permanent molars deemed of poor prognosis in a Class I malocclusion.

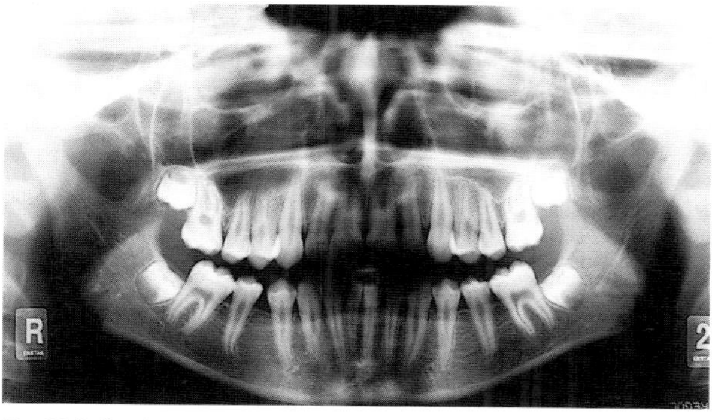

**Fig. 34** Following the removal of first permanent molars in Fig. 33 (no appliance therapy).

# 7 / Mixed dentition IV

## Labial segment problems

### Upper median diastema

*Aetiology*

Normal development, which usually reduces as 3|3 erupt; midline supernumerary; absent or small 2|2 (Fig. 35); incisor proclination; generalised spacing condition. Maxillary frenum may contribute if the arch is spaced; look for blanching of incisive papilla on stretching the frenum and notching between 1|1 on radiograph.

*Investigations*

Maxillary anterior occlusal radiograph if there is a large diastema to exclude the presence of a supernumerary.

*Management*

- Wait until 3s erupt as the diastema may reduce.
- Remove supernumerary unless it is well above the apices of 1|1.
- Fixed appliance to close the diastema; bonded retention with build up of 2|2 if they are small.

### Dilaceration

*Definition*

Sudden angular alteration in the long axis of the crown or in the root of a tooth (Fig. 36).

*Aetiology*

*Trauma*: most commonly follows the intrusion of a; it is often accompanied by enamel and dentine hypoplasia.
*Developmental*: characteristic labial and superior coronal deflection of the affected tooth.

*Management*

*Surgical removal* if dilaceration is moderate/severe. *Surgical exposure/orthodontic alignment* is occasionally possible if dilaceration is mild and the apex is destined not to perforate the cortical plate.

### Traumatic loss of 1

*Management*

*Immediate*: reimplantation or fitting of URA with a replacement tooth to prevent centreline shift and tilting of the adjacent teeth (Fig. 37).
*Later*: consider autotransplantation of a premolar, or adhesive bridgework if the reimplantation is unsuccessful.

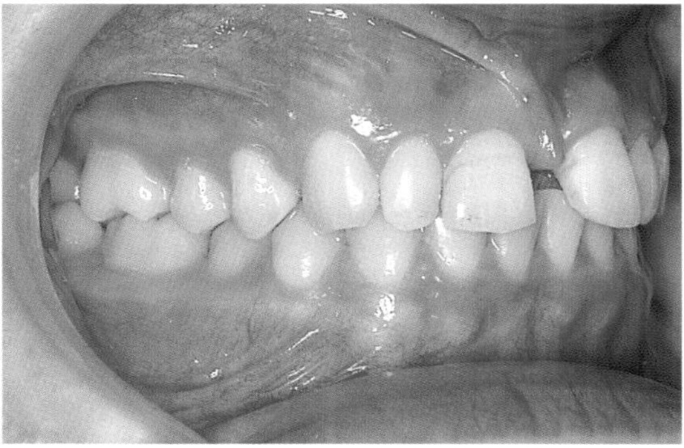

**Fig. 35** Upper median diastema with small 2|2 and low frenal attachment.

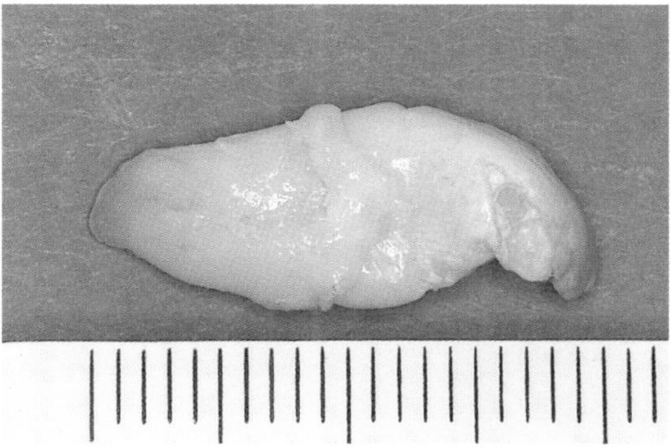

**Fig. 36** Dilacerated and hypoplastic |1.

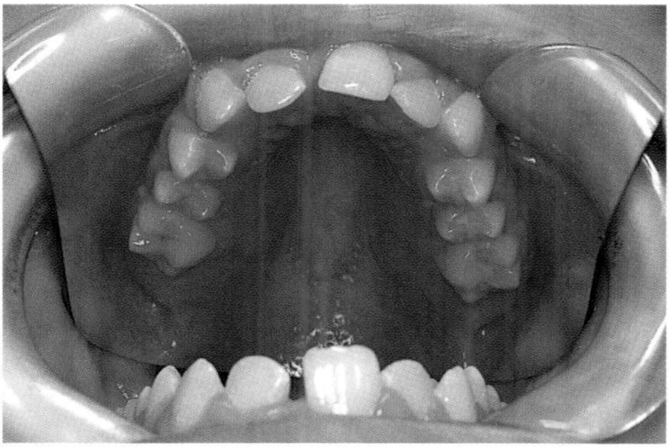

**Fig. 37** Tilting of the adjacent teeth after the loss of 1|.

### Retained primary incisor

*Aetiology and management*

See under 'retained primary tooth' (p. 23), 'mesiodens' (p. 19), and below.

### Incisors in crossbite

*Aetiology*

See page 53.

*Management*

Remove the retained primary incisor if it is deflecting the eruption of its permanent successor (Fig. 38). If there is accompanying mandibular displacement and a positive overbite is attainable (Fig. 39), URA with a Z-spring to the offending incisor usually suffices. The removal of $\underline{c}$s may be required to facilitate crossbite correction of $\underline{2}$, or of $\overline{c}$s to allow lingual movement of a labially-placed lower incisor (Fig. 22a, b; p. 18).

### Finger/thumb-sucking habits

*Effects*

Depending on the positioning of the finger(s) or thumb, and the frequency and intensity, the habit may procline upper incisors, retrocline lower incisors, increase the overjet (often asymmetrically), reduce the overbite, or lead to crossbite tendency of the buccal segments (Fig. 40).

*Management*

Gentle persuasion to discontinue the habit is usually best.

### Early correction of increased overjet

*Management*

Consider an initial phase of functional appliance therapy (see pp. 67–70) if there is marked risk of incisor trauma, but fixed appliances (see pp. 63–66) with or without extractions are often necessary at a later stage.

*Disadvantages*

Treatment may be prolonged and patient cooperation may wane. There is a slight risk of resorption of incisor roots if they are retracted into the eruption path of $\underline{3}$s.

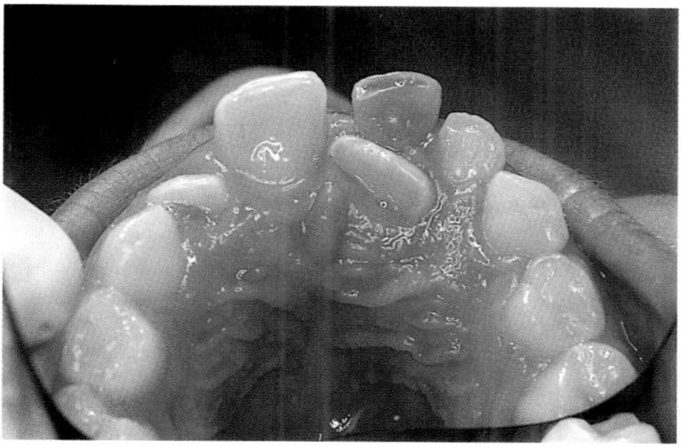

**Fig. 38** Retained |a deflecting |1.

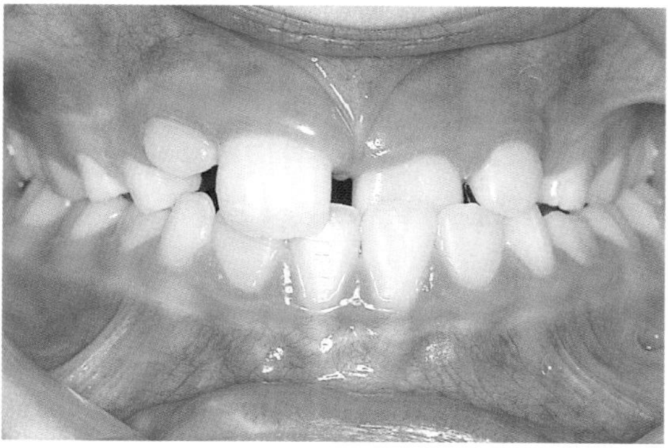

**Fig. 39** |1 crossbite with associated mandibular displacement.

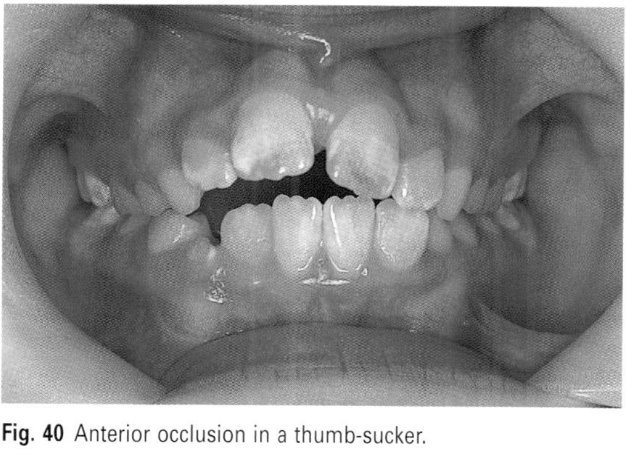

**Fig. 40** Anterior occlusion in a thumb-sucker.

## Ectopic maxillary canines

*Prevalence*

About 2% of the Caucasian population have ectopic maxillary canines (15% buccal; 85% palatal); occasionally $\underline{3}$ is transposed with $\underline{4}$ or $\underline{2}$ (the former is more common).

*Aetiology*

- The longest eruption path of any permanent tooth.
- Buccal displacement is more common in a crowded arch (Fig. 41).
- Palatal displacement is more common in an uncrowded arch and is associated with small, absent or abnormal root formation of $\underline{2}$s (Fig. 42a, b) and Class II Division 2 malocclusion.

*Detection*

*Clinical*: buccal and palatal palpation; observe the inclination of $\underline{2}$ (it will be labially inclined if $\underline{3}$ is high and buccal or low and palatal).

*Radiographic*: dental panoramic tomograph (DPT) is useful in the initial assessment but requires a standard occlusal view (Fig. 42a, b) or two periapicals taken with a tube shift to aid localisation by parallax. Assess the axial inclination, the apex location, the vertical and mesiodistal position relative to the incisor roots, and the root length of $\underline{c}$.

*Management (buccal canine)*

As the arch is usually crowded, remove $\underline{4}$ as $\underline{3}$ is starting to erupt (Fig. 41) to expedite spontaneous alignment. If $\underline{3}$ is mesially inclined, alignment may require a buccal canine retractor on URA; a fixed appliance is required if $\underline{3}$ is upright or distally inclined.

If there is severe crowding with $\underline{2}$ and $\underline{4}$ in contact, consider the removal of $\underline{3}$.

If eruption of $\underline{3}$ is delayed and the position favourable for alignment, consider surgical exposure of $\underline{3}$ with apically repositioned or replaced flap with bonded attachment or magnet to facilitate alignment.

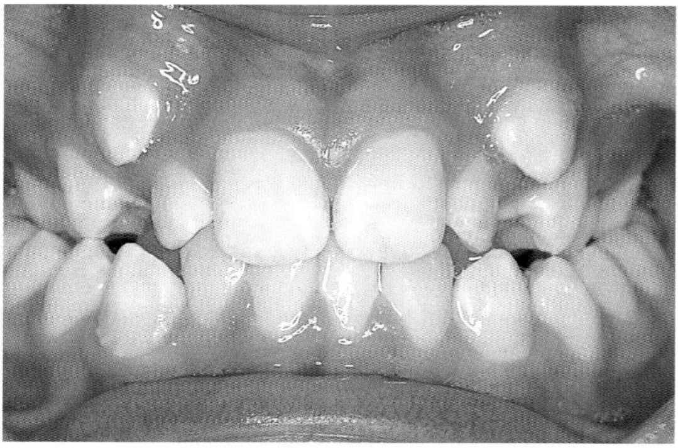

**Fig. 41** Buccal $\underline{3}$s in a crowded arch; note the mesial inclination of $\underline{3}$s.

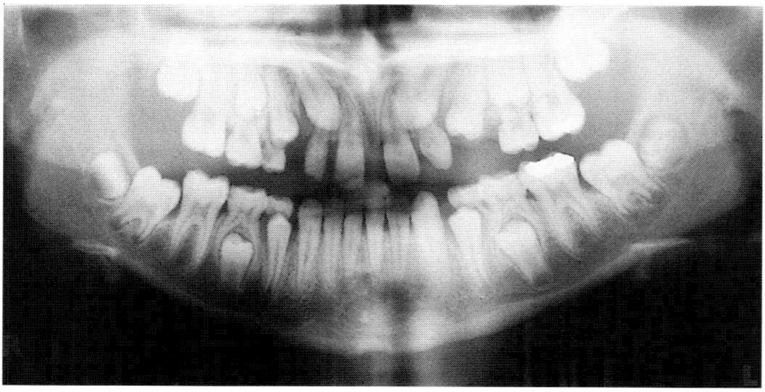

**Fig. 42a** DPT of 42b.

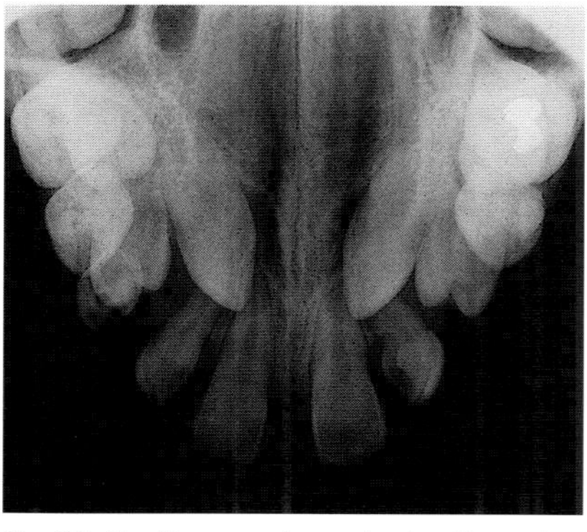

**Fig. 42b** Maxillary anterior occlusal radiograph of Fig. 42a shows $\underline{3|3}$ palatal; note the spacing and small $\underline{2|2}$.

*Management (palatal canine)*

- Remove c: in mixed dentition, if the arch is uncrowded and 3 is mildly displaced, extraction of c may allow the successful eruption of 3.
- Retain c and review the position of 3 radiographically to ensure that there is no cystic change or resorption of adjacent teeth. Prosthetic replacement of c is required when it is eventually lost.
- Exposure of 3 requires a well disposed patient, and good oral hygiene and dentition. For exposure to be successful, 3 should overlap ≤ half width of 1 and be no higher than ≥ apex 2; the root apex of 3 should not be distal to 5 and its long axis to the mid-sagittal plane should be ≤ 30°; the arch should be spaced or it should be possible to create space. A fixed appliance is required to align the apex of 3.
- Transplantation: consider if the prognosis for the alignment of 3 is hopeless, there is adequate space in the arch for 3, intact removal of 3 is possible, and there is adequate buccal/palatal bone. The prognosis is improved if 3 root is two-thirds formed, there is minimal handling at surgery, and rigid splinting is avoided. Five year survival rate is around 70%.
- Removal of 3: if the patient is not keen for appliance therapy, 2 and 4 are in contact, or there is good root length on c and the aesthetics of c are acceptable (Fig. 43).
- Retain 3: occasionally in a young patient unsure about treatment but who may elect to proceed with alignment of 3 later. Monitor the status of 3 and the incisor roots with an annual radiographic examination.

*If there is incisor resorption.* (Fig. 44) Removal of 3 may arrest resorption but if resorption is extensive, removal of the incisor may be unavoidable, allowing 3 to erupt.

*If 3 is transposed.* (Fig. 45) Assess if the root apices are completely or partially transposed, assess the degree of crowding and malocclusion type. It may be necessary to accept the transposition, extract the most displaced tooth, or align the arch.

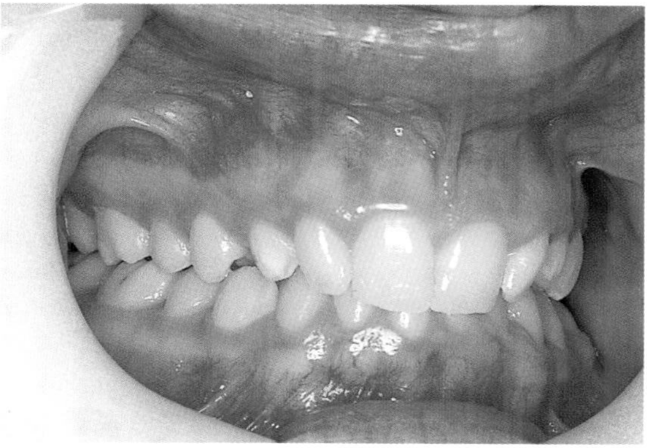

Fig. 43 Acceptable occlusion with c| retained; 3| was removed. The patient did not want appliance therapy.

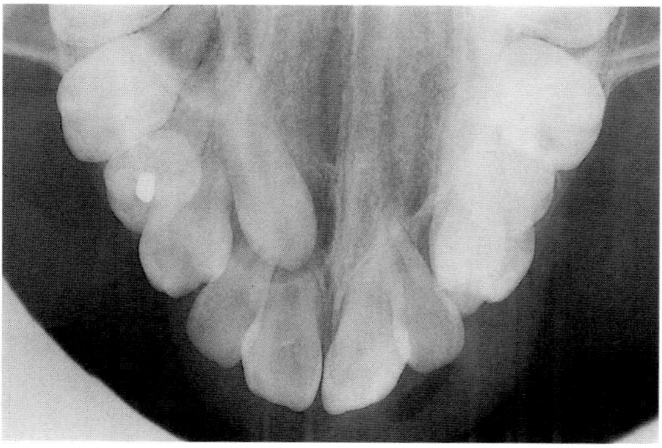

Fig. 44 Resorption of 21| by 3|.

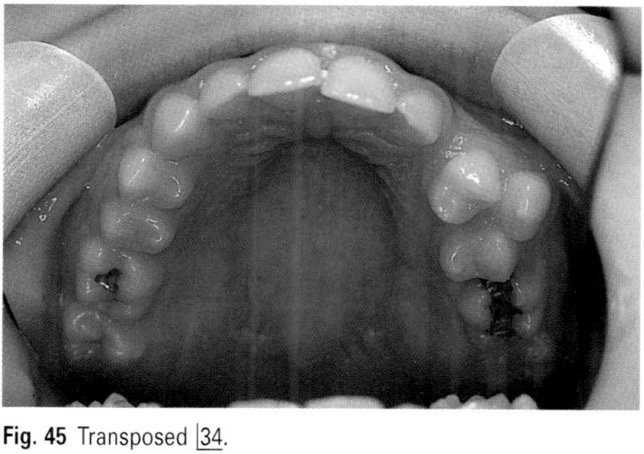

Fig. 45 Transposed |34.

# 8 / Class I malocclusion

*Incidence*

50–55% of Caucasians.

*Aetiology*

*Skeletal.* Class I, Class II or Class III malocclusion with incisor compensation for any underlying skeletal discrepancy. Lower facial height (LFH) may be increased or a mild transverse skeletal discrepancy may exist.

*Soft tissues.* Not prime aetiological factors except in bimaxillary proclination where labial movement of incisors (Fig. 46) may result from tongue pressure in the presence of unfavourable lip tone.

*Dental.* Tooth/dental arch discrepancy leading to crowding (Fig. 47) or spacing (Fig. 48) is the principal cause. Early loss of primary teeth, large or small teeth, supernumerary or absent teeth also influence inherent dentoalveolar disproportion.

*Occlusal features*

- Class I incisor relationship.
- Variable molar relationship depending on whether mesial drift has followed any extractions.
- Crowding is often concentrated in $\underline{3}$, $\overline{5}$ areas.
- Occasional crossbite with associated mandibular displacement and centreline shift.

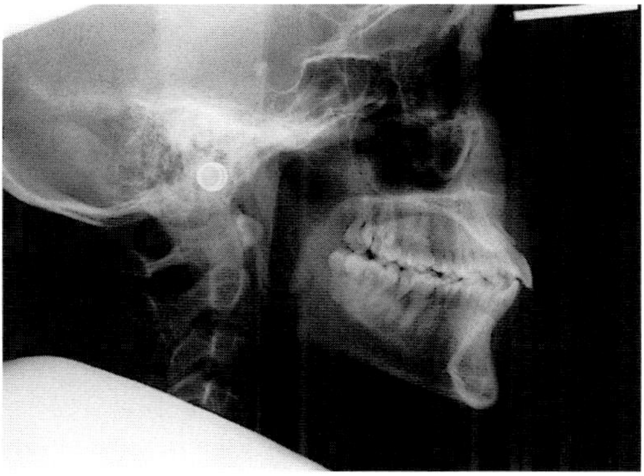

**Fig. 46** Bimaxillary proclination.

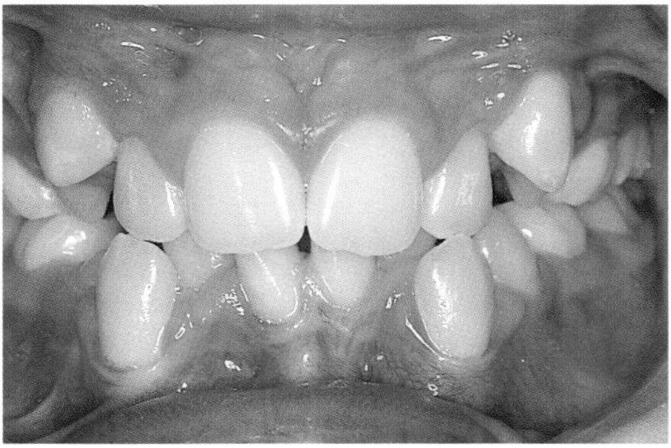

**Fig. 47** Class I malocclusion with crowding.

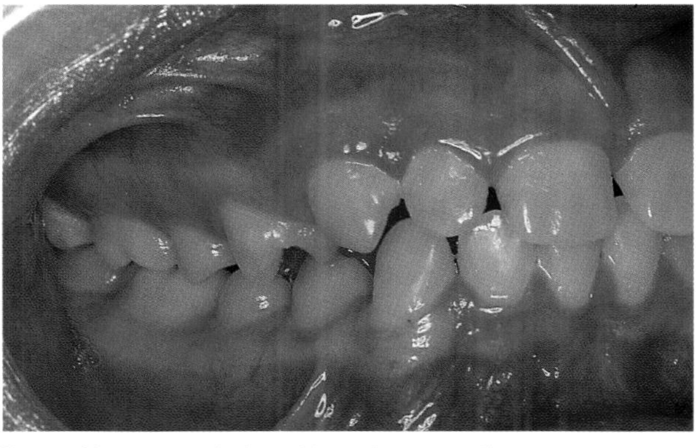

**Fig. 48** Class I malocclusion with spacing; 2s small.

## Treatment

*Crowding*

*Some basic guidelines for Class I cases*:

- Mild crowding is best accepted (Fig. 49).
- Moderate crowding usually requires first premolar extractions; maximal alignment of incisors and canines is likely in the first 6 months post extraction when 3s are mesially tilted and there are no occlusal interferences.
- Severe crowding is often managed expediently by the removal of most displaced teeth or by the extraction of more than one tooth per quadrant. Anchorage planning is critical (Fig. 50a, b).
- Late lower labial segment crowding is common in mid to late teens. It is best accepted if it is mild. If the posterior occlusion is Class I and the arches are aligned with slight overbite increase and moderate to severe crowding, consider the extraction of one or two lower incisors followed by fixed appliance alignment and bonded retention.

*Bimaxillary proclination*

Proclination of upper and lower incisors is seen typically in people of African origin, but may also occur in Caucasians with Class I, Class II Division 1, or Class III malocclusion. Overjet is increased in Class I cases due to incisor angulation. Incisor retraction is generally unstable unless the lips have good muscle tone and become competent with treatment – otherwise permanent retention is indicated.

*Spacing*

Spaced dentition is generally rare in Caucasians. It results from a disproportion in the size of the teeth relative to the arch size, or from the absence of teeth. When spacing is mild, acceptance is usually best, or consider composite additions or porcelain veneers to increase the mesiodistal width of the labial segment teeth. If spacing is more marked, orthodontic treatment to localise spacing at specific sites may be necessary prior to fitting a prosthesis or to implant placement.

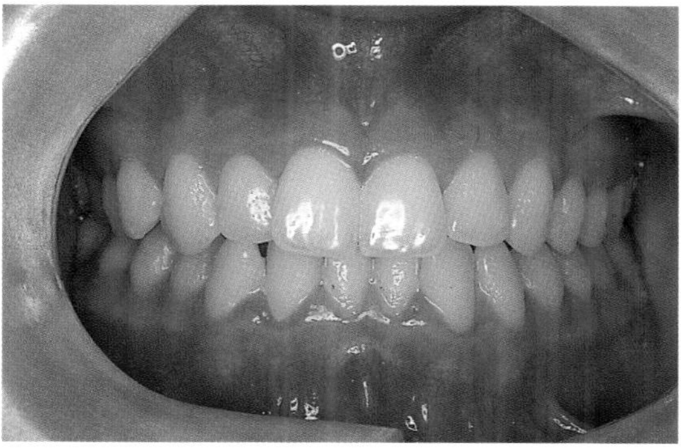

**Fig. 49** Class I malocclusion with acceptable mild crowding.

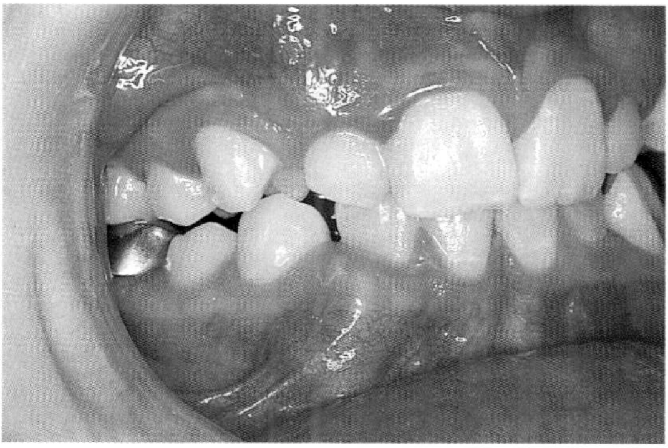

**Fig. 50a** Class I malocclusion with severe crowding (note lingual arch in place).

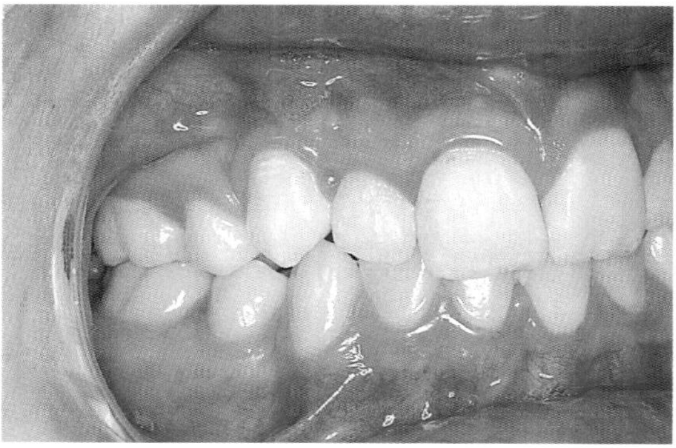

**Fig. 50b** Following URA/lingual arch space maintenance only and removal of 4s (note lower centreline shift accepted).

# 9 / Class II Division 1 malocclusion

*Incidence*

15–20% of Caucasians.

*Aetiology*

*Skeletal.* Usually Class II (mandibular deficiency primarily; Fig. 51a) but may be Class I or mildly Class III. Anterior vertical facial proportions vary.

*Lips, tongue and habits.* In general, the greater the Class II skeletal pattern, the greater the likelihood of the lips being incompetent (Fig. 51a) and with a reduced lower facial height, an anterior oral seal may be produced by the lower lip lying under the upper incisors. By proclining the upper and to a lesser degree retroclining the lower incisors, the overjet is worsened. A hyperactive lower lip (Fig. 51b) may increase an overjet by retroclining $\overline{21|12}$. With an increased lower facial height, an anterior oral seal is often produced by forward positioning of the tongue, tending to reduce the overbite and compensate for the Class II discrepancy by proclining the lower incisors. Rarely, a primary atypical swallowing pattern is present. For the effects of digit or thumb-sucking habit see page 29.

*Crowding.* Labial displacement of upper or lower incisors may, respectively, aggravate or ameliorate an overjet.

*Occlusal and related characteristics*

- Overjet is increased with possible trauma to $\underline{1|1}$ (Fig. 51c) (the risk doubles with an overjet $>$9 mm, also there is greater risk in boys than in girls and where the lips are incompetent).
- Overbite varies from complete and traumatic to incomplete to anterior open bite.
- Molars are usually Class II provided there is no mesial drift from early loss of primary teeth.
- If lips are grossly incompetent, drying of the upper labial gingivae may worsen an established gingivitis.

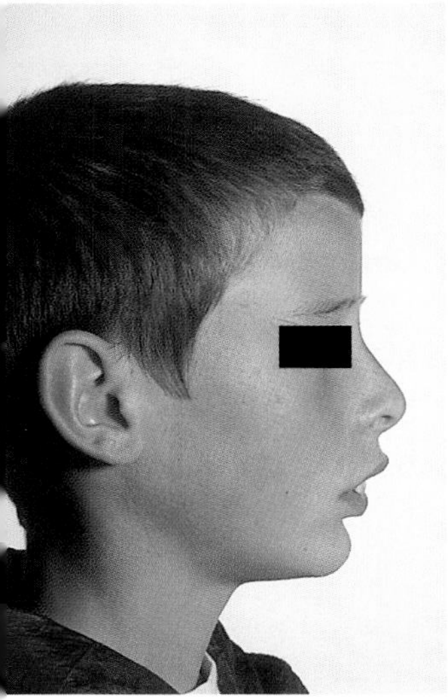

1a Class II skeletal pattern with
petent lips.

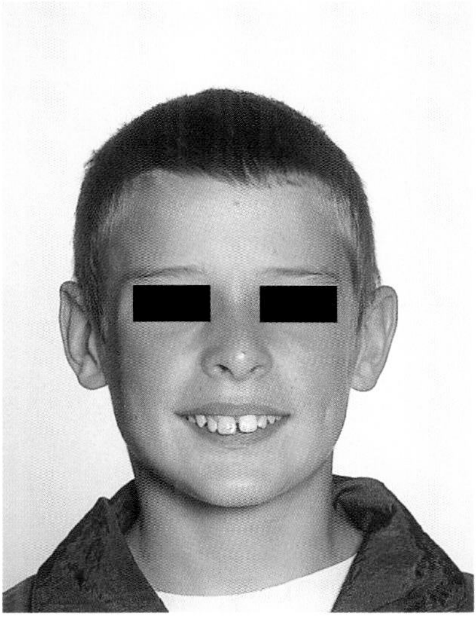

**Fig. 51b** Expressive lower lip acting under 21|12.

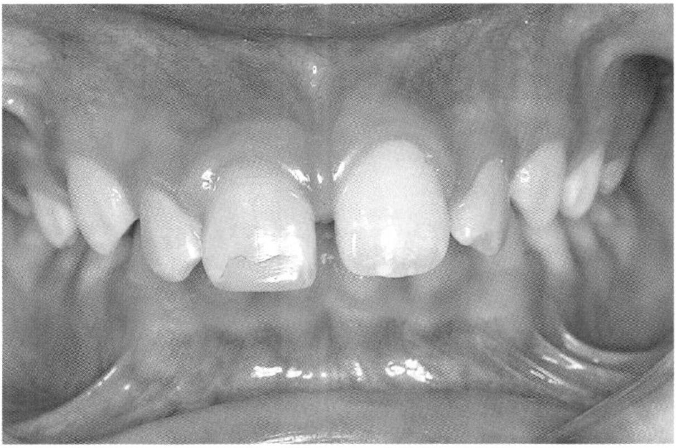

**Fig. 51c** Associated Class II Division 1 malocclusion; trauma to 1|.

## Treatment

Consider the patient's age, skeletal pattern, pattern of mandibular growth, form and relationship of lips and tongue at rest and in function, and space requirements (Fig. 52a, c).

*Class I or mild Class II skeletal pattern*

*Consider URA* where FMPA slightly reduced/average; there are no unfavourable soft tissue factors (e.g. grossly incompetent lips or primary tongue thrust); the lower arch is uncrowded, acceptably aligned or moderately crowded with $\overline{3|3}$ mesially inclined and no incisor rotations; $\underline{3|3}$ mesially inclined; $\underline{21|12}$ aligned and proclined so that after tipping to reduce overjet, the likely final inclination is not $\leq 95°$ to the maxillary plane; the patient is growing, which facilitates overbite reduction.

*Fixed appliance is indicated* particularly if the inclination of canines and maxillary incisors is not amenable to tipping; rotations are present; intrusion of incisors is required for overbite reduction; and space closure is desired (Fig. 52c, d).

*Moderate Class II skeletal pattern*

*Growth modification.* This is only possible just before and during the pubertal growth spurt using a functional appliance (see pp. 67–70), headgear, or both.

*Orthodontic camouflage.* This usually involves the extraction of $\underline{4|4}$ and fixed appliances to bodily retract upper incisors. It is only acceptable where a Class II skeletal pattern is no worse than moderate, vertical facial proportions are good, and arches are well aligned.

*Orthognathic surgery.* This is indicated where there is a marked Class II skeletal pattern with considerably reduced or increased facial proportions and/or a gummy smile in an adult.

*Retention and post-treatment stability*

Provided the interincisal angle is within the normal limits, overjet is completely reduced with the upper incisors in soft tissue balance (Fig. 52b, d) (i.e. no tongue thrust and the lower lip covering at least the incisal third of the upper incisors): a few months of retention will often suffice, but retention until growth is complete is required following functional appliance therapy.

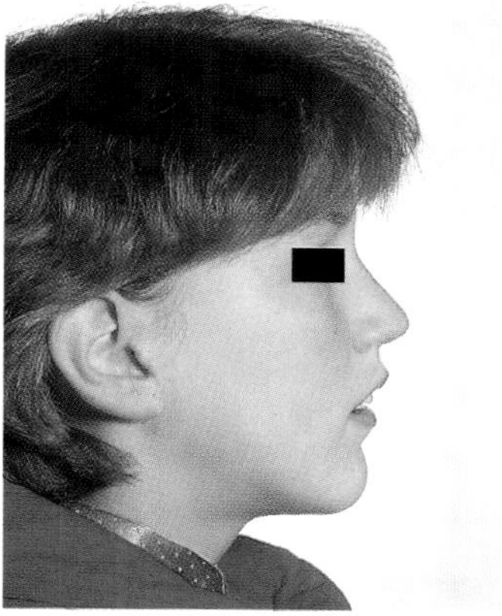

**Fig. 52a** Profile pre-treatment.

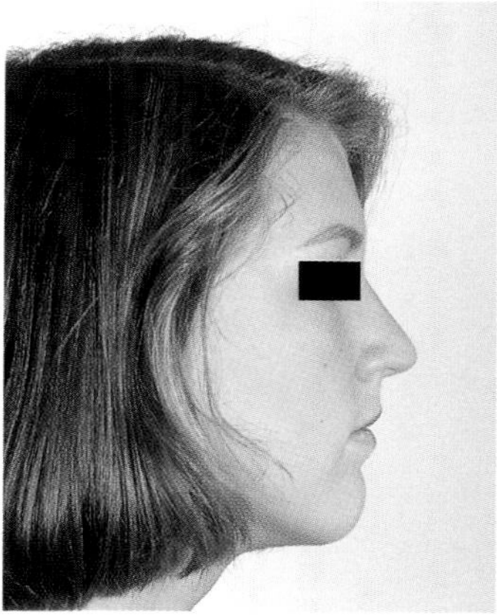

**Fig. 52b** Profile post-treatment.

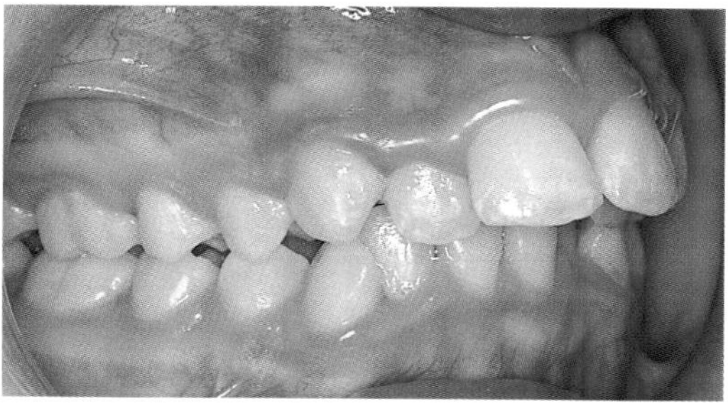

**Fig. 52c** Class II Division 1 malocclusion; note mildly proclined 1|1; bodily displaced 2|2.

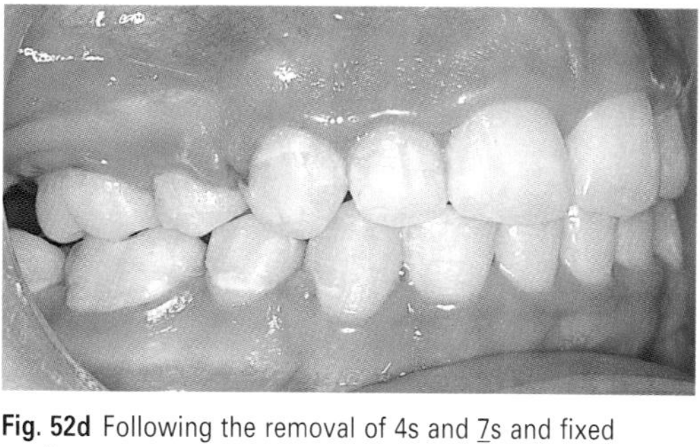

**Fig. 52d** Following the removal of 4s and 7s and fixed appliance treatment.

# 10 / Class II Division 2 malocclusion

*Incidence*

10% of Caucasians.

*Aetiology*

*Skeletal pattern.* Usually mildly Class II but may be Class I or mildly Class III; reduced FMPA associated with anterior mandibular growth rotation which tends to increase overbite; a relatively wide maxillary base may lead to buccal crossbite of premolars.

*Soft tissues.* Lips are usually competent with a high lower lip line. If the lower lip is also hyperactive, bimaxillary retroclination will result.

*Dental.* Often a poorly developed cingulum on the upper incisors and occasionally an acute crown/root angulation. Crowding is worsened by retroclination of incisors.

*Occlusal features*

- Typically $\underline{1|1}$ retroclined; $\underline{2|2}$ proclined and mesiolabially rotated; overbite is deep and complete; overjet is minimal/slightly increased (Fig. 53).
- Occasionally $\underline{21|12}$ and $\overline{21|12}$ retroclined with $\underline{3|3}$ buccal (Fig. 54).
- Overbite may be traumatic (Fig. 55).
- Mild Class II buccal segment relationship with possible buccal crossbite of $\underline{4|4}$ (Fig. 54) or $\underline{54|45}$.

*Treatment planning principles*

Beware of lower arch extractions only, as a deep overbite may become traumatic as the lower labial segment drops lingually.

Some proclination of $\overline{21|12}$ and mild lower intercanine expansion is often possible and stable, thereby providing space for overbite reduction and the relief of crowding.

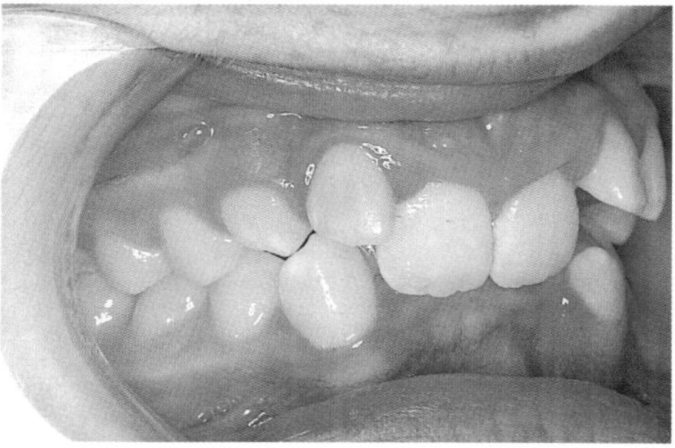

**Fig. 53** Typical Class II Division 2 malocclusion.

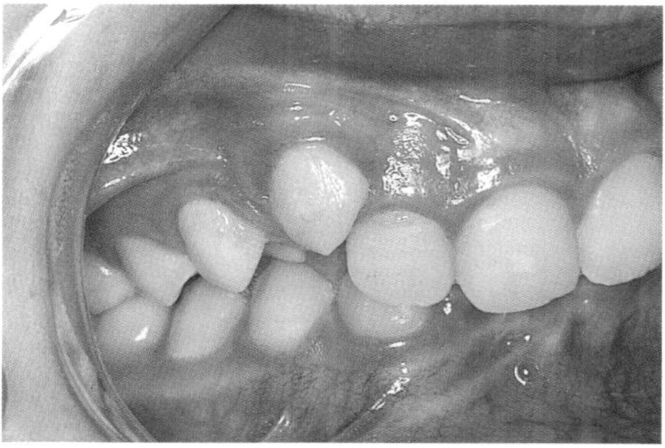

**Fig. 54** 21|1 retroclined; 3| buccal; buccal crossbite 4|.

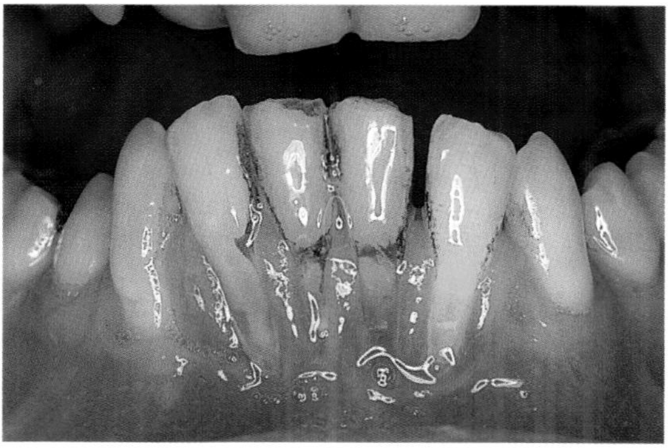

**Fig. 55** Traumatic overbite.

## Treatment

*Class I or mild Class II skeletal pattern*

*Where overbite and retroclination of $\underline{1|1}$ or $\underline{21|12}$ are to be accepted.* Confine treatment to the relief of upper arch crowding and upper labial segment alignment.

*If lower arch acceptable, upper arch mildly crowded with at most half unit Class II molar relationship.* Consider moving the upper buccal segment distally with headgear (which may require the removal of $\underline{7|7}$), followed by canine retraction just sufficient for labial segment alignment. Extraction of $\underline{5|5}$ and fixed appliance therapy is an alternative where cooperation with headgear is unlikely. If buccal segment relationship is a full unit Class II, or extraction of $\overline{5|5}$ is required for the relief of crowding, removal of $\underline{4|4}$ is usually indicated.

*Where overbite and retroclination of $\underline{1|1}$ or $\underline{21|12}$ to be corrected.* Indicated where the overbite is deep and complete on gingival or palatal tissues with existing or potential trauma. Fixed appliances are required to effect overbite reduction by the proclination of lower incisors alone or in combination with palatal/lingual torque (Fig. 56a, b). Extractions are required if lower arch crowding is severe; distal movement of buccal segments or extractions provide space for the correction of the incisor relationship in the upper arch. Reduce the interincisal angle to ≤135° for the best prospect of stable correction.

*More marked Class II skeletal discrepancy*

*Growth modification.* This is indicated in a growing child with ideally a well-aligned lower arch. Procline $\underline{1|1}$ or $\underline{21|12}$ and then use a functional appliance. To detail occlusion, may then require fixed appliances (Fig. 57a, b).

*Orthognathic surgery.* This is indicated in an adult patient particularly if an overbite is deep and traumatic.

*Post-treatment stability*

Alignment of $\underline{2|2}$ and overbite reduction are prone to relapse. Bonded retention is advisable for $\underline{2|2}$. Flat anterior bite plane on URA retainer is recommended until growth is complete to promote overbite stability.

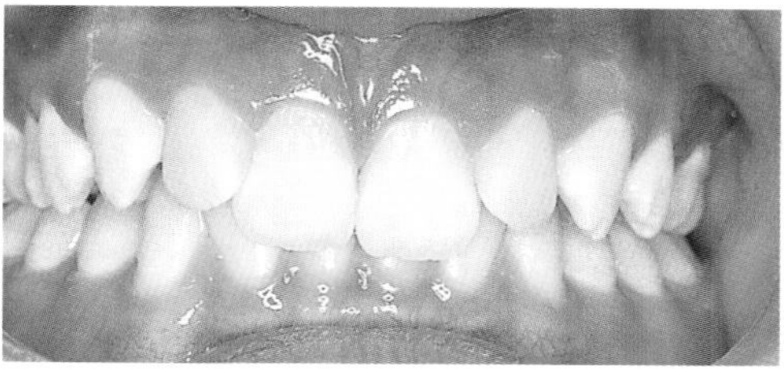

**Fig. 56a** Pre-treatment.

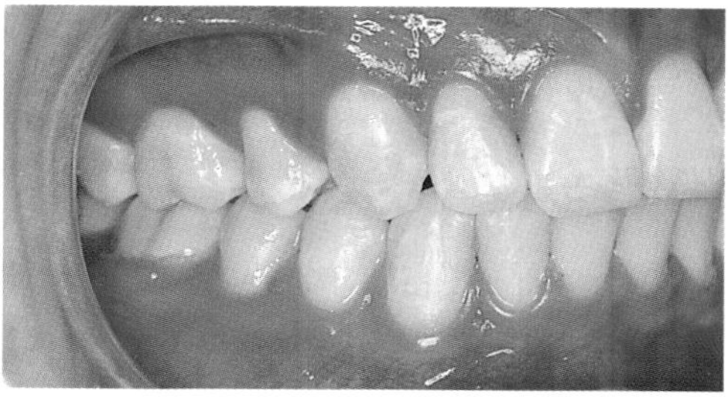

**Fig. 56b** Following the extraction of 4s and fixed appliance therapy.

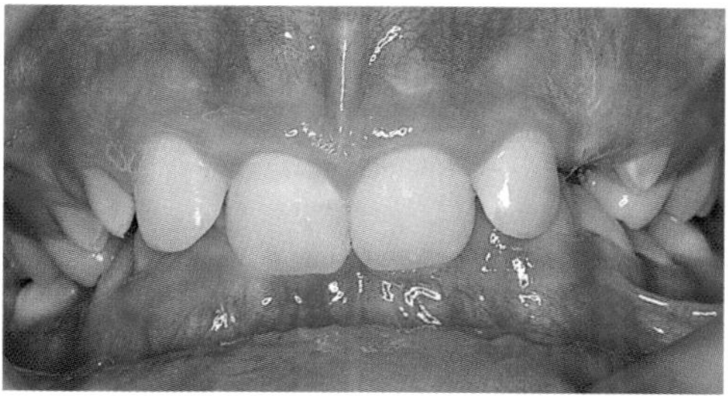

**Fig. 57a** Pre-treatment.

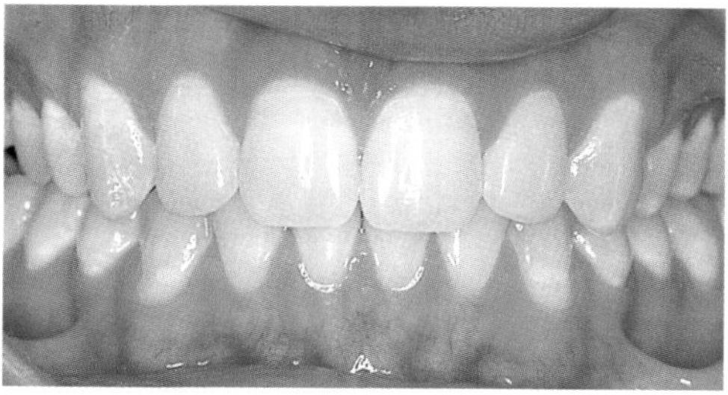

**Fig. 57b** After functional followed by fixed appliance therapy.

# 11 / Class III malocclusion

*Incidence*

3% of Caucasians.

*Aetiology*

*Skeletal pattern.* Usually Class III associated with a long mandible, forward placement of the glenoid fossa positioning the mandible more anteriorly (Fig. 58), short and/or retrognathic maxilla, short anterior cranial base or a combination of these (Fig. 59); it may be Class I with Class III incisor relationship due to incisor position or inclination. FMPA may be reduced/average/increased. There is commonly a transverse discrepancy with a narrow maxillary and a wider mandibular base but worsened by a Class III skeletal pattern.

*Soft tissues.* Where lips are competent, dentoalveolar compensation (proclination of $\underline{21|12}$; retroclination of $\overline{21|12}$) to mask the severity of skeletal pattern is likely; if FMPA is increased and lips are incompetent with anterior open bite, $\overline{21|12}$ may be proclined.

*Dental.* As the upper arch is often narrow and short, crowding is more common and more severe than in the lower arch (Fig. 60).

*Occlusal features*

Class III incisor relationship

- Frequently $\underline{21|12}$ proclined; $\overline{21|12}$ retroclined.
- Upper arch crowding is common; lower arch more commonly aligned or spaced.
- Crossbites of labial and/or buccal segments are common; a crossbite may be associated with mandibular displacement.

*Treatment planning*

Consider the degree of anteroposterior and vertical skeletal discrepancy, the potential direction and extent of future facial growth, incisor inclinations, the amount of overbite, the ability to achieve edge-to-edge incisor relationship, and the degree of upper and lower arch crowding. The prognosis is usually more favourable where the skeletal pattern is mildly Class III with average to low FMPA, deep overbite, upper arch crowding, proclined lower incisors, and the ability to achieve an edge-to-edge incisor relationship exists.

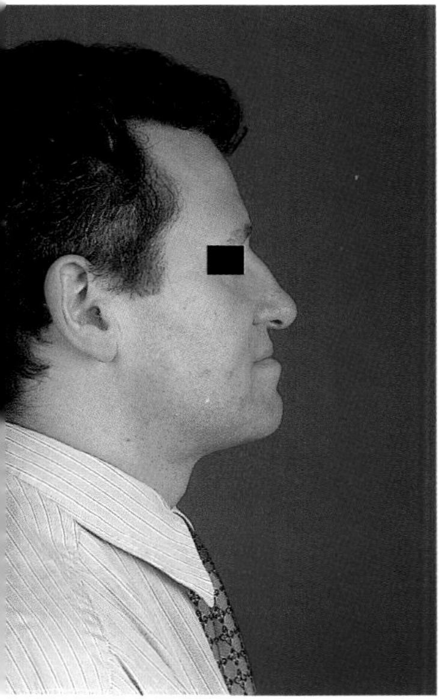

8 Mandibular prognathism.

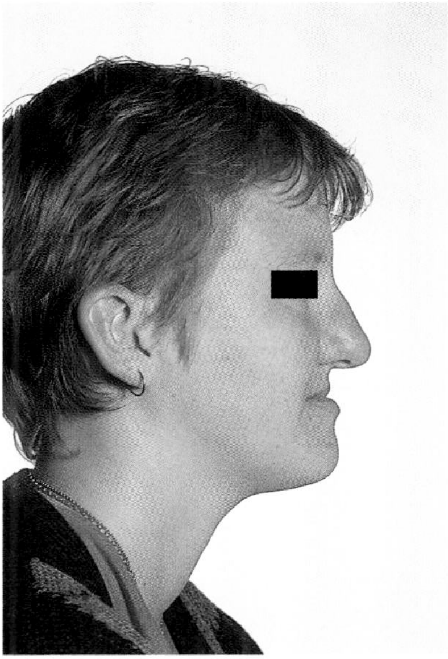

**Fig. 59** Maxillary retrognathism and mild mandibular prognathism.

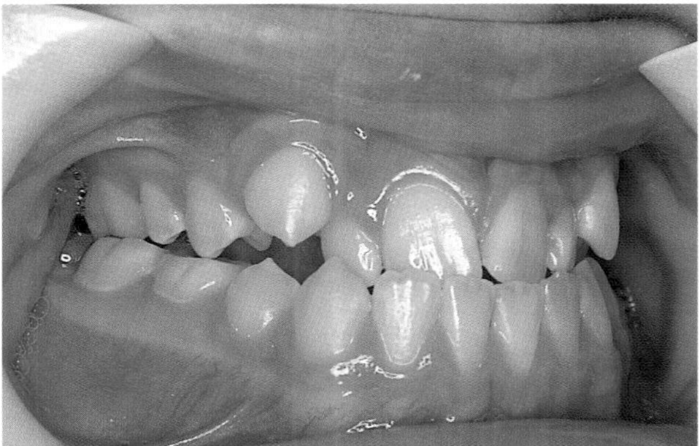

**Fig. 60** Class III malocclusion; uncrowded lower arch/moderately crowded upper arch (note the mild dentoalveolar compensation).

## Treatment

*Accept*

When the skeletal pattern is mildly Class III and/or incisor relationship is acceptable with minimal crowding and no mandibular displacement.

*Normal or mild Class III skeletal pattern*

*If overbite is reduced,* accept the incisor relationship and align teeth with possible extractions. Delay upper arch extractions until after crossbite correction as space will be forthcoming from arch expansion.

*If overbite is normal or increased* with upright upper incisors, consider proclination of $\underline{21|12}$. This is best undertaken in early mixed dentition before $\underline{3|3}$ move labial to $\underline{2|2}$ roots; otherwise wait until $\underline{3|3}$ retracted before proclining $\underline{2|2}$. Use URA with screw or Z-spring and posterior capping, but a fixed appliance may be required for the correction of other occlusal anomalies. Reassess the need for upper arch extractions after the correction of anterior crossbite. Distal movement of upper buccal segments is not favoured as it restrains maxillary growth. Removal of $\overline{c|c}$ in early mixed dentition (Fig. 22a, b; p. 18) or of $\overline{4|4}$ in permanent dentition may allow the lower labial segment to drop lingually and increase the overbite.

*Mild to moderate Class III skeletal pattern*

Where the overbite is average or increased.

*Growth modification* by reverse pull headgear attached to a maxillary splint or Frankel III (Fig. 61). Attempts to modify growth are generally disappointing as there is an inherent tendency for growth to be unfavourable. Also retention is prolonged.

*Orthodontic camouflage.* Aim to correct the incisor relationship by retroclination of the lower labial segment and/or proclination of the upper labial segment. Extraction of $\overline{4|4}$ is usually necessary with Class III intermaxillary traction to upper and lower fixed appliances (Fig. 62a, b). Consider the use of reverse pull headgear to an upper fixed appliance to aid proclination of $\underline{21|12}$. Extract in the lower arch only where the likelihood of successful overjet correction is favourable. Avoid the extrusion of upper molars as this reduces overbite.

*Severe Class III skeletal pattern*

Either align arches and accept the incisor relationship or resort to orthognathic surgery.

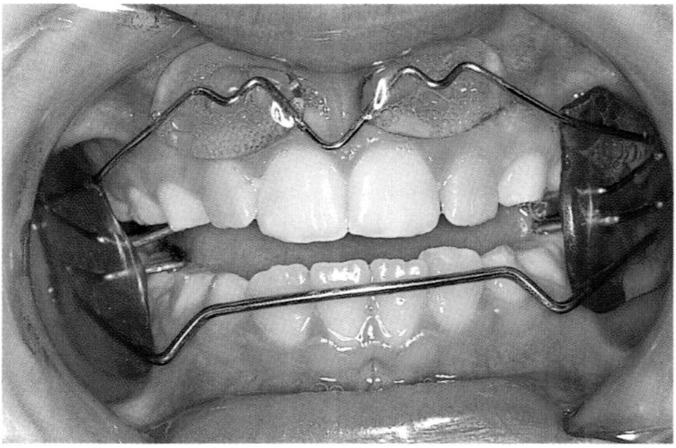

**Fig. 61** Frankel III appliance.

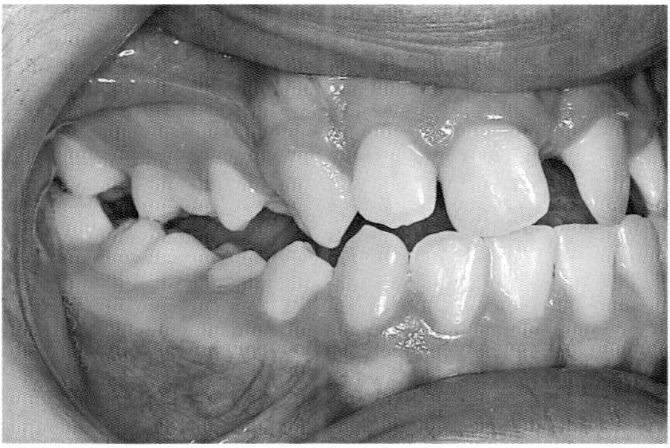

**Fig. 62a** Pre-treatment ($\underline{5|5}$ absent).

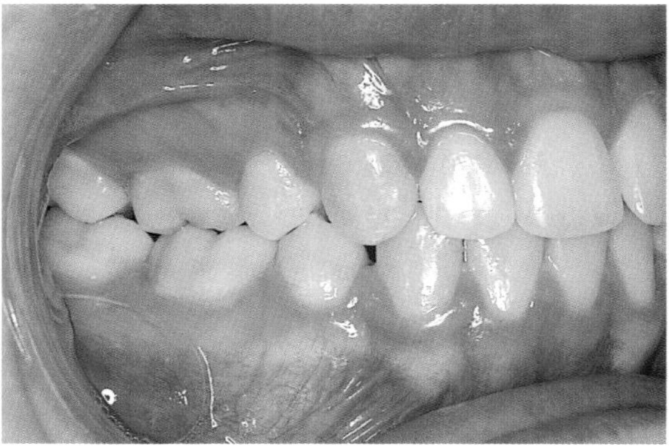

**Fig. 62b** After removal of $\overline{4}$s and fixed appliance therapy.

# 12 / Crossbite

*Definition*

Buccolingual malrelationship of upper and lower teeth.

*Classification*

Anterior or posterior (unilateral or bilateral) with or without mandibular displacement.

*Buccal crossbite.* Lower teeth occlude buccal to corresponding upper teeth (Fig. 63).

*Lingual crossbite (scissors bite).* Lower teeth occlude lingual to palatal cusps of upper teeth (Fig. 64).

*Aetiology*

One or more of the following may be implicated:

*Skeletal.* Mismatch in the widths of the dental arches or an anteroposterior skeletal discrepancy – lingual crossbite is common in Class II cases (Fig. 64); buccal and/or anterior crossbite occurs often with Class III malocclusion (Fig. 63). Rarely, growth restriction of the mandible following condylar trauma or condylar hyperplasia is implicated.

*Soft tissue.* With a digit-sucking habit, the tongue is lowered and cheek contraction during sucking is unopposed, displacing the upper posterior teeth into buccal crossbite.

*Crowding.* Where inherent crowding exists, $\underline{2}$ may be displaced palatally (Fig. 65) and $\underline{7}$ or $\underline{8}$ pushed into scissors bite.

*Local causes.* Retention of a primary tooth or early loss of $\underline{e}$ in a crowded arch may lead to crossbite of the successor.

*Treatment need*

If there is associated mandibular displacement, crossbite may predispose to temporomandibular joint dysfunction syndrome in susceptible individuals; displacing anterior occlusion may compromise lower incisor periodontal support (Fig. 22a; p. 18).

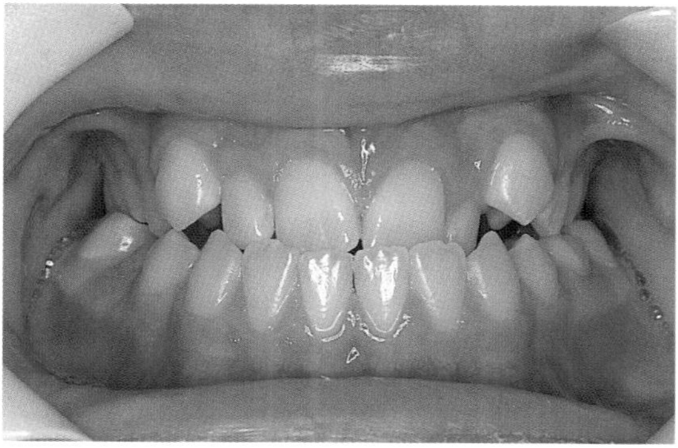

**Fig. 63** Bilateral buccal crossbites and anterior crossbite; Class III malocclusion.

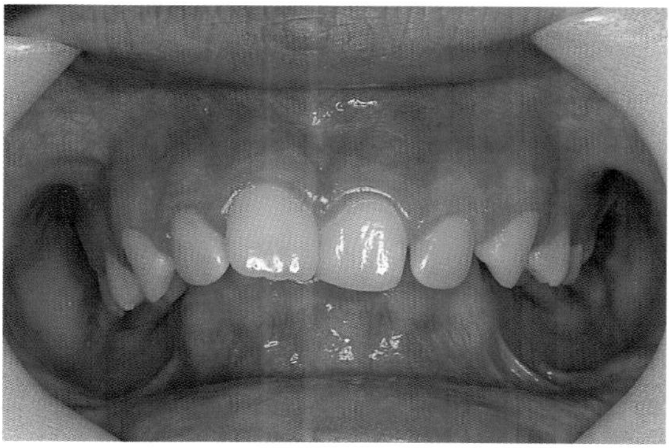

**Fig. 64** Bilateral lingual crossbite; Class II Division 1 malocclusion.

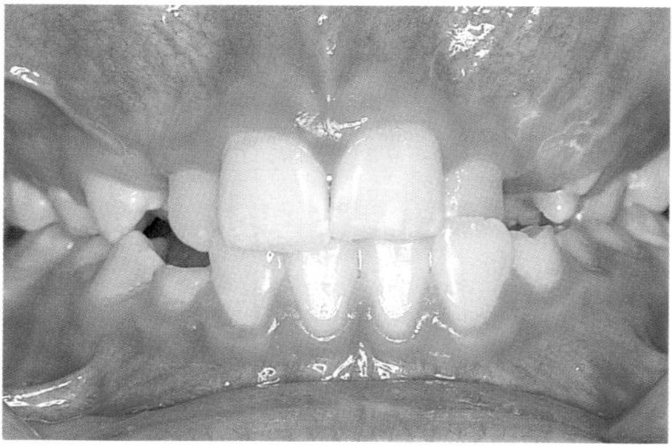

**Fig. 65** $\underline{2}$s in crossbite in a crowded arch.

## Treatment

*Anterior crossbite*

If one or two incisors are in crossbite, mandibular displacement usually exists. Correct early in mixed dentition if adequate overbite is likely (Fig. 22a, b; p. 18). Extractions may be needed to allow tooth alignment.

If tooth inclination is amenable to tipping, use URA with buccal capping to free the occlusion and Z-spring for proclination (Fig. 66), or consider a screw section clasping the teeth to be moved. If insufficient overbite is likely or an incisor is bodily displaced, use a fixed appliance in the permanent dentition. For correction of two or more incisors see page 49.

*Unilateral buccal crossbite*

For crossbite correction of a premolar or molar, consider the use of a T-spring or screw section, respectively, on an URA.

If reciprocal movement of opposing teeth is required, use fixed attachments and cross elastics. Consider also the relief of crowding if a tooth is mildly displaced, or extraction of a tooth in crossbite if there is more marked displacement.

For correction of unilateral buccal segment crossbite associated with a mandibular displacement, use an URA with a midline expansion screw and buccal capping or quadhelix (Fig. 67), provided teeth are not tilted buccally.

If there is unilateral buccal segment crossbite with no mandibular displacement, as there is no functional problem, correction is not usually indicated unless it is part of a more comprehensive treatment in cases of cleft palate or condylar hyperplasia.

*Bilateral buccal crossbite*

Usually accept, as a functional problem is rare. Rapid maxillary expansion (Fig. 68) of the mid-palatal suture can be tried, but no later than early teenage years. As half of the dental expansion is lost, some overexpansion is advisable.

*Lingual crossbite*

Where a single tooth is displaced due to crowding, it can often be corrected by its extraction or by alignment with the buccally approaching arm on an URA once space has been created.

*Complete unilateral*

*With displacement.* Use fixed appliances to expand lower arch/contract upper arch. Stability is likely if good buccal intercuspation has been achieved.

*Complete unilateral*

*No displacement.* Consider surgery.

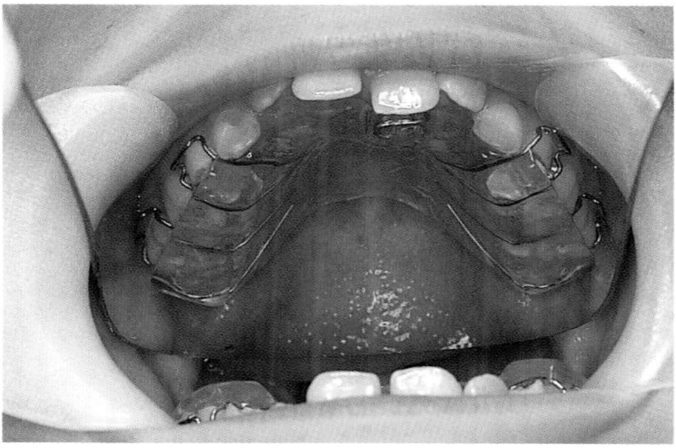

**Fig. 66** URA to procline $\lfloor\underline{1}$.

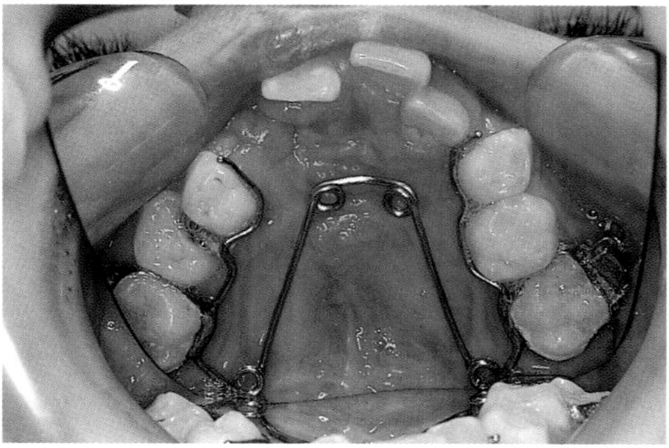

**Fig. 67** Quadhelix appliance.

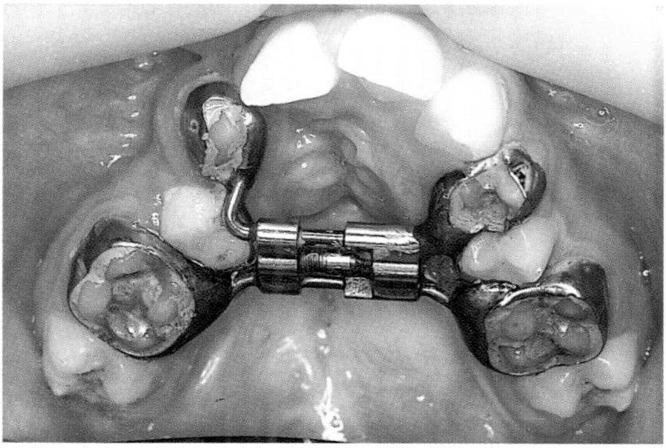

**Fig. 68** Hyrax screw for rapid maxillary expansion (note the repaired cleft palate).

# 13 / Anterior open bite (AOB)

*Definition*

Incisors do not overlap vertically when posterior teeth are in occlusion (Fig. 69).

*Aetiology*

A combination of any/all of the following:

*Skeletal pattern.* Increase in lower anterior face height and steep FMPA. May be worsened by downward and backward pattern of mandibular growth.

*Soft tissues.* Rarely endogenous tongue thrust; usually with an associated lisp and some incisor proclination.

*Habits.* Persistent digit-sucking habit (Fig. 40; p. 30) often produces asymmetric AOB.

*Localised failure of alveolar development.* Observed in clefts of lip and alveolus but may have no known cause in other cases.

*Treatment*

Unless AOB is due to a habit, treatment is complex:

*Accept.* If AOB is mild, or where the prospect of stability is poor due to adverse skeletal and/or soft tissue factors, notably grossly incompetent lips and/or suspicion of endogenous tongue thrust – relieve crowding and align arches only.

*Habit breaker.* URA or modified palatal arch.

*Growth modification.* High pull headgear to upper molars in mild cases or to posterior/full coverage maxillary splint or functional appliance with buccal capping if there is a Class II pattern and more marked AOB.

*Camouflage.* Occasionally incisor retraction following relief of crowding (Fig. 70a, b) is stable if the lips become competent post-treatment. It is essential to avoid mechanics which will worsen AOB (e.g. cervical headgear, intermaxillary elastics to molars).

*Surgery.* If AOB is severe, consider surgery when growth is complete. Stability is often doubtful.

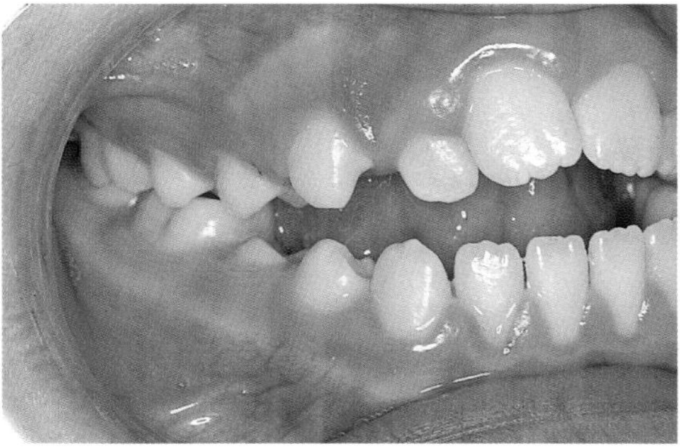

**Fig. 69** Anterior open bite due to increased FMPA.

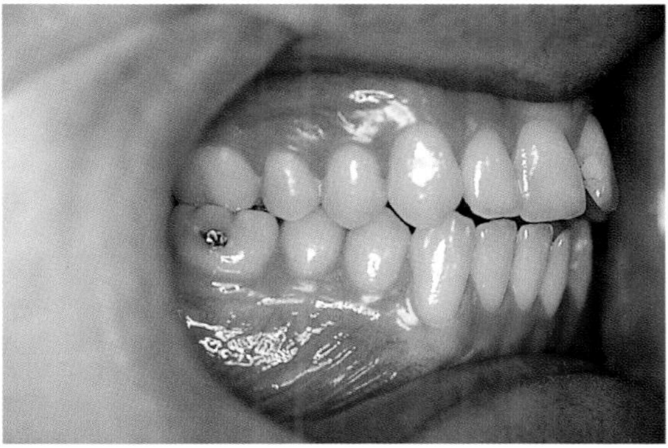

**Fig. 70a** Pre-treatment.

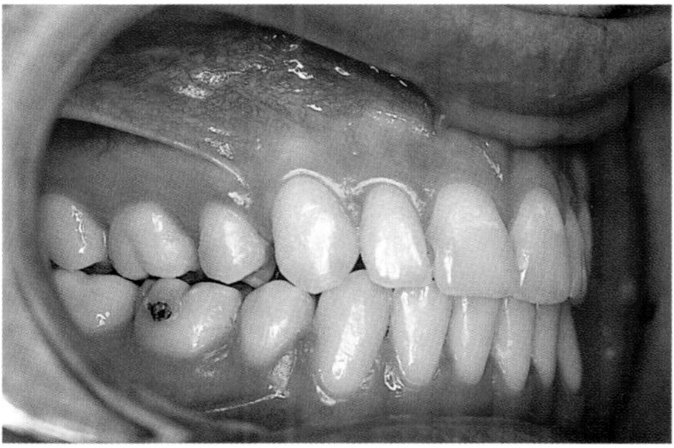

**Fig. 70b** Following removal of 4s and fixed appliance therapy.

# 14 / Removable appliances

*Definition*

An appliance removable from the mouth consisting primarily of wire and acrylic components. It may be active or passive and is used almost exclusively in the upper arch. Also most functional appliances are removable (see pp. 67–70).

*Indications*

Tilting of teeth; for space maintenance in mixed/early permanent dentition; to help transmit forces to groups of teeth (e.g. arch expansion or distal movement of buccal segments); to free the occlusion and facilitate crossbite correction or other tooth movement; for overbite reduction in a growing child; when minor rotation of an incisor or extrusion and rotation (with a fixed attachment) is required; as a retainer following removable or fixed appliance treatment.

## Active component

*Springs* (Figs 71 & 72). Force (F) $\propto dr^4/l^3$ where d = deflection of spring, r = radius of wire, l = length of spring. With 0.5 mm palatal finger spring, 3 mm activation is likely to produce appropriate force (0.3 N); with 0.7 mm spring, 1 mm of activation is adequate.

*Bows* (Fig. 71). Mechanically more complex than springs; Roberts retractor (Fig. 73) offers good flexibility and a favourable stability ratio.

*Screws.* Act directly on a tooth or via the baseplate. They make an appliance bulky (see Fig. 75; page 60). They exert large intermittent forces but they are tolerable due to small (0.2 mm) activation with each turn.

*Elastics.* The tooth to be moved and the distance over which the elastic is to be stretched determine the choice of elastic. Elastics should be changed daily. Avoid use of elastics for overjet reduction as they slide up the teeth, flatten the arch and may produce gingival recession.

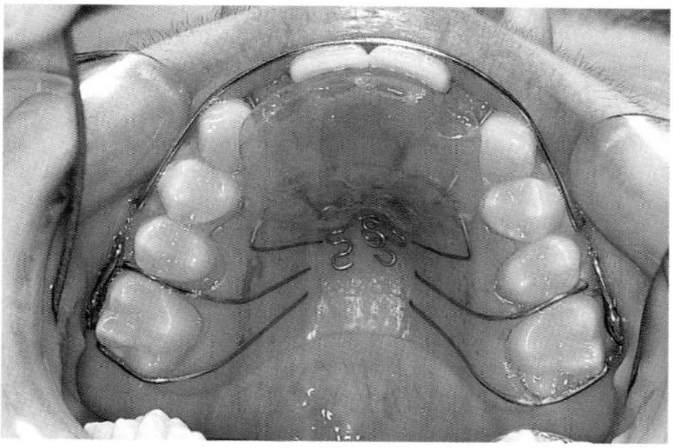

**Fig. 71** Palatal finger springs; long labial bow.

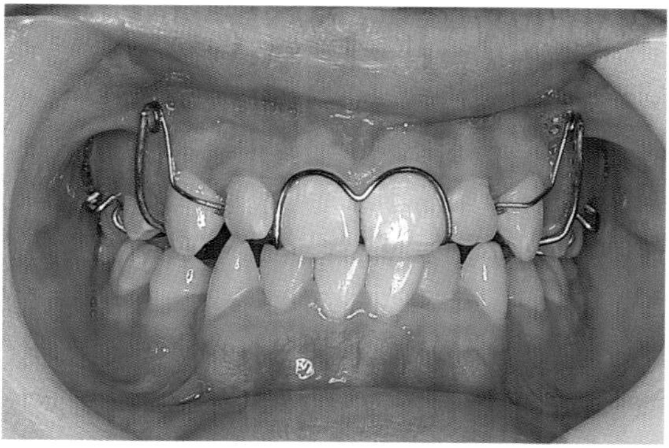

**Fig. 72** Buccal canine retractors.

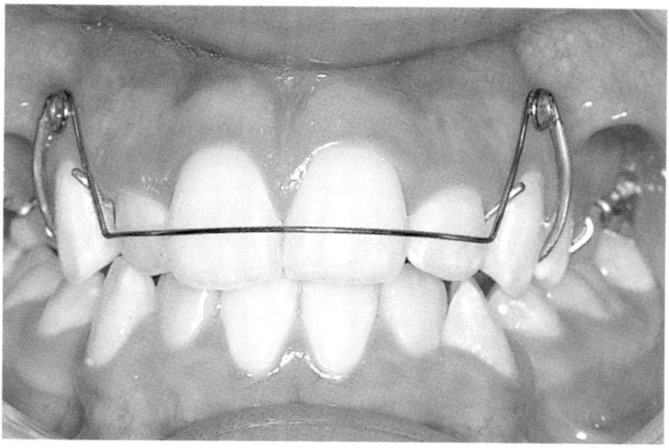

**Fig. 73** Roberts retractor.

## Retention component

Some commonly used means are:

*Adams clasp.* Used posteriorly in the arch (Figs 74, 75, 76). Arrowheads engage about 1 mm of mesial and distal undercuts on the tooth. 0.7 mm wire is used for molars; 0.6 mm wire is advisable for premolars and primary molars. The clasp is easily modified to incorporate hooks for elastics, or tubes may be soldered for extraoral anchorage (Fig. 75).

*Southend clasp.* Recommended anteriorly with 'u' loop engaging the undercut between incisors (Fig. 74).

*Long labial bow.* 0.7 mm wire (0.8 mm if it includes reverse loops). This is useful in preventing buccal drifting of teeth during mesial or distal movement (Fig. 71; p. 58); it can also be fitted to the teeth as a retainer.

## Baseplate

This is usually made of cold-cured acrylic but may be heat-cured. It connects the other components; guards palatal springs; aids anchorage by contact with the palate and with teeth intended not to move; and transfers active component forces to the anchorage. It may also be active.

*Flat anterior biteplane (FABP).* Used to reduce overbite (Fig. 74) or to remove occlusal interference to allow tooth movement. FABP should contact two or three lower incisors.

*Posterior bite platform.* To remove occlusal interferences and to facilitate tooth movement when overbite reduction is unnecessary. It is commonly used in the correction of unilateral buccal crossbite with displacement or incisor crossbite (Fig. 76).

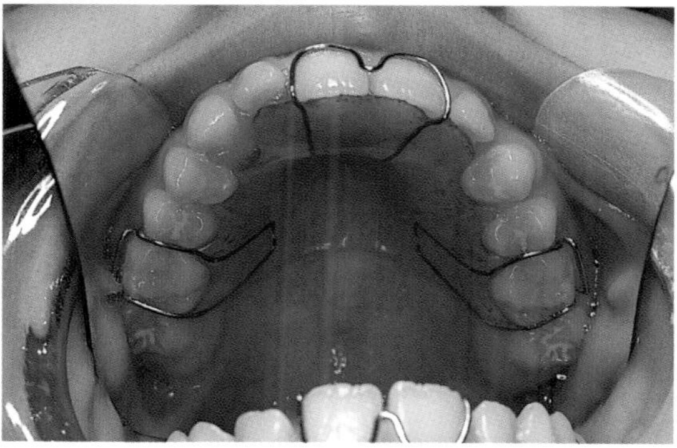

**Fig. 74** Southend and Adams clasps; flat anterior biteplane.

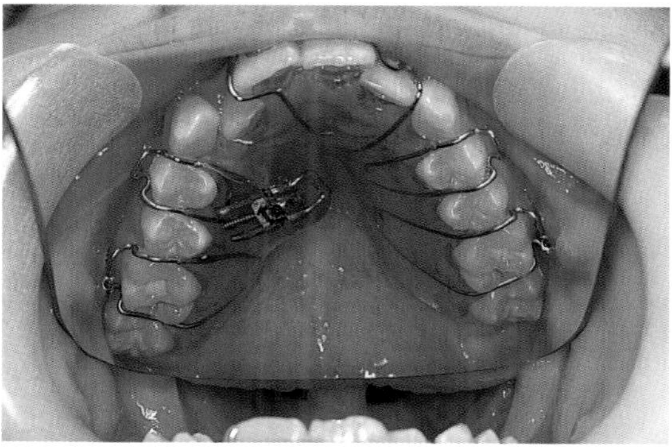

**Fig. 75** Tubes soldered to 6|6 clasps; screw to move the right buccal segment distally.

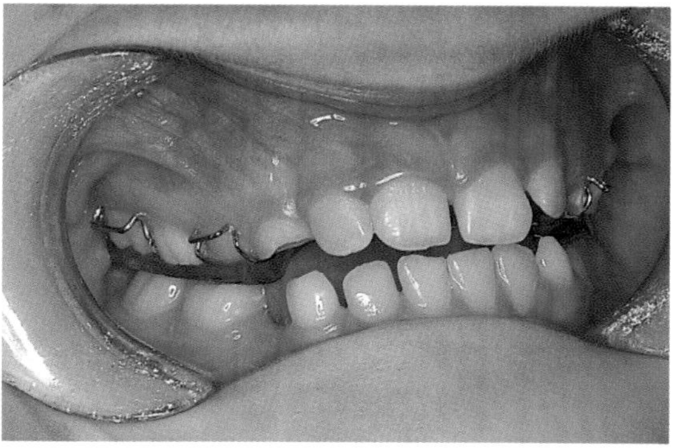

**Fig. 76** Posterior capping to facilitate crossbite correction on 1|.

# 15 / Anchorage

*Definition*

Resistance to the force of reaction generated by the active components. It is best thought of in terms of available space for intended tooth movement.

*Tendency for anchorage loss is related to:*

*Force applied.* Bodily movement is more anchorage demanding than tipping movement.

*Root surface area (RSA).* Teeth with a larger RSA or a block of teeth with a large RSA will resist anchorage loss more than those with a smaller RSA.

*Mesial drift tendency.* This is greater in the upper than in the lower arch, and will be worse if URA is left out.

*FMPA.* Space loss is easier with increased than with reduced FMPA.

*Occlusal interdigitation.* Where this is good, mesial drift is less likely.

*To minimise anchorage loss*

Use force as light as possible for the intended tooth movement (about 30–50 g for tipping; about 150–250 g for bodily movement), move the minimum number of teeth at one time, and increase the resistance of the anchor teeth.

*Reinforcing anchorage intraorally*

*Intramaxillary*: incorporate the maximum number of teeth in the same arch in the anchorage unit.

*Mucosal coverage*: URA is better than a fixed appliance.

*Intermaxillary*: use teeth in the opposing arch. Suitable with fixed appliances – Class II (Fig. 77) or Class III (Fig. 78) traction.

*Reinforcing anchorage extraorally*

*By headgear* (Fig. 79): to URA or fixed appliance. Anchorage requires 200–250 g for 10 h/day; extraoral traction requires 500 g for 14–16 h/day.

*Headgear safety*

Fit two safety mechanisms, preferably a facebow with locking device (e.g. Nitom™) and a safety release spring mechanism attached to the headcap (Fig. 79). Issue verbal and written safety instructions to both patient and parents and check the headgear at each visit.

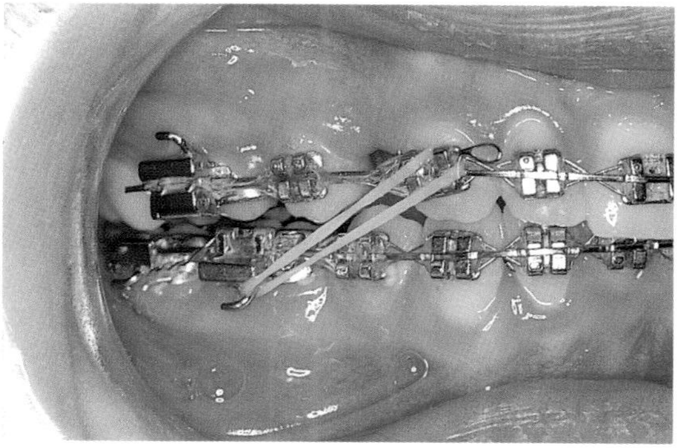

**Fig. 77** Class II traction.

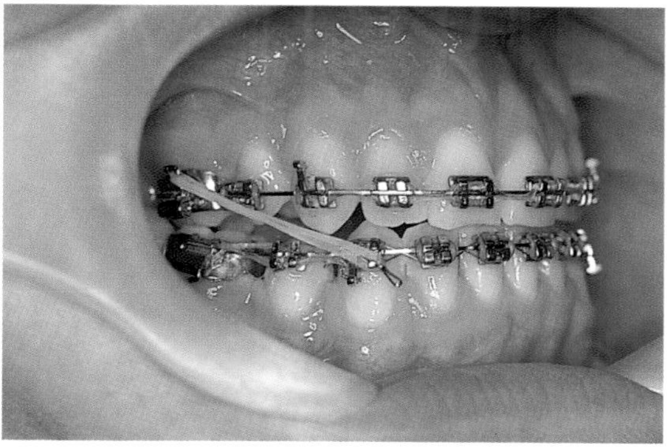

**Fig. 78** Class III traction.

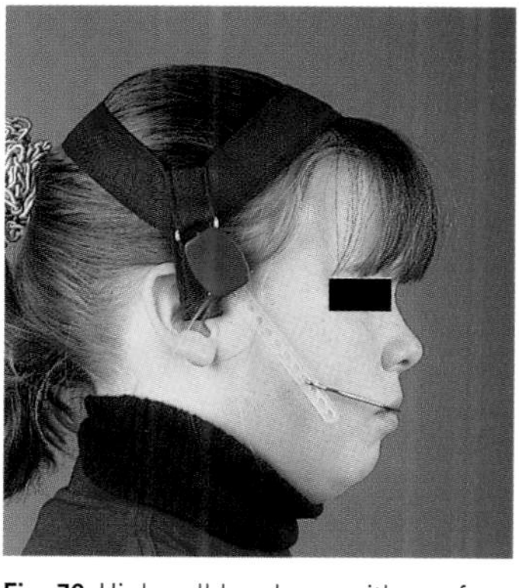

**Fig. 79** High pull headgear with a safety mechanism on the headcap.

# 16 / Fixed appliances

*Definition*

An appliance fixed to teeth by attachments through which force application is by archwires or auxiliaries.

*Components*

*Brackets and bands* (Fig. 80). Brackets (bonded to teeth, by acid etch/composite resin or alternative system) allow the teeth to be directed by active components (archwires and/or accessories). Bands are cemented to molars or used when repeated bond failure occurs.

*Archwires.* These may be round or rectangular. Usually, round active wire is used initially (Fig. 81); rectangular passive wire with auxiliaries is used later in treatment (Fig. 80).

*Auxiliaries.* Elastics or elastomeric modules/chain/thread (Figs 80, 81); springs.

*Indications for fixed appliances*

Bodily movement, particularly of incisors to correct mild to moderate skeletal discrepancies; overbite reduction by incisor intrusion; correction of rotations (Fig. 81); extensive lower arch treatment; alignment of grossly misplaced teeth, particularly those requiring extrusion; closure of spaces; multiple tooth movements required in either one or both arches.

*Appliance management*

Cooperative patient with excellent oral hygiene; adjustment visits at 4–6-week intervals.

*Anchorage control*

Bodily rather than tipping movement places greater strain on the anchorage. Reinforce anchorage by bonding more teeth and ligating them together; palatal (Fig. 82) or lingual arches; intermaxillary traction; extraoral means.

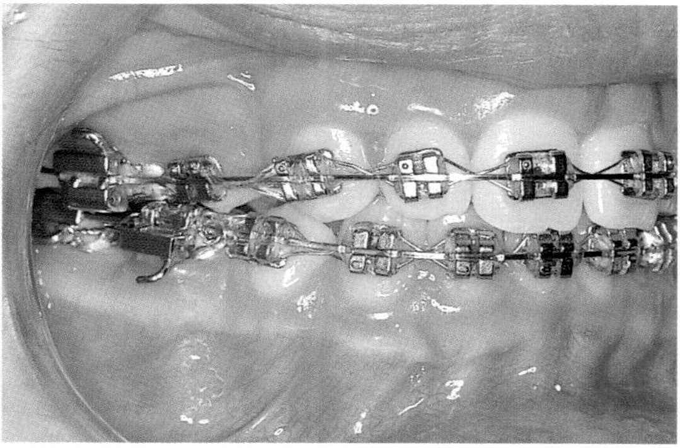

**Fig. 80** Fixed appliances, rectangular archwires, elastomeric modules and chain.

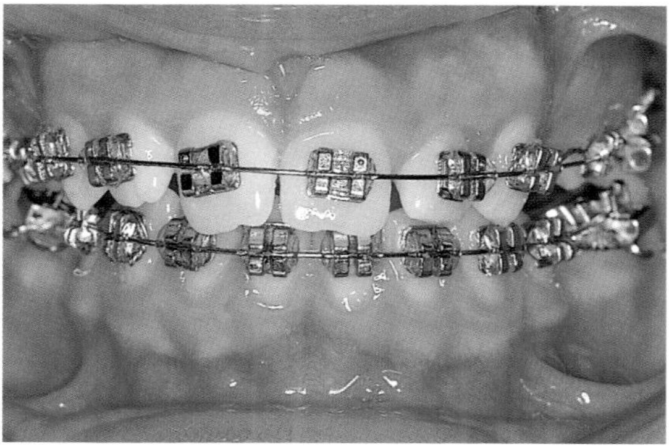

**Fig. 81** Initial aligning round wires.

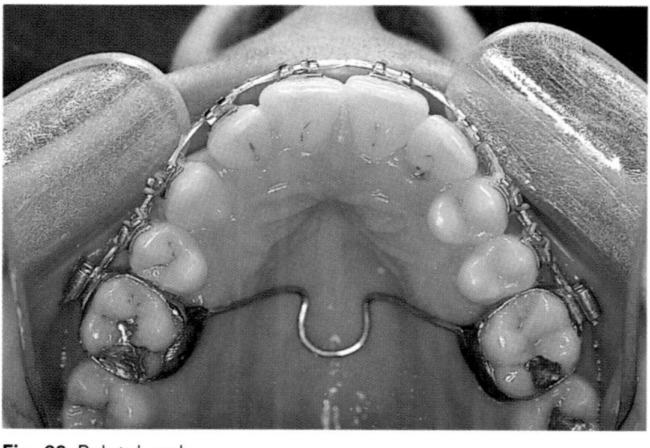

**Fig. 82** Palatal arch.

## Appliance types

### Most common pre-adjusted appliances

*Edgewise.* Uses an individual bracket with a rectangular slot for each tooth to give it 'average' inclination and angulation and to allow placement of flat archwires. Bracket prescriptions described by Andrews (Fig. 83) and Roth are available.

*Tip-edge.* Based on the Begg philosophy but the narrow brackets also have preadjusted values to allow the placement of rectangular wires in the final stages of treatment (Fig. 84).

### Lingual appliance

Uses brackets bonded to the lingual/palatal surfaces of the teeth and specially configured archwires. Aesthetic, but uncomfortable for the patient and difficult to adjust.

### Sectional appliance

Components are attached to teeth in (usually) one segment of the arch, normally for localised alignment as part of adjunctive treatment, especially in adults (see Fig. 92; p. 72).

### Fixed – removable

URA with bands cemented to $\underline{6}$s for extraoral traction (Fig. 85); bracket bonded to a rotated incisor and whip spring hooked to labial bow for derotation; bracket bonded to a favourably inclined palatal canine and traction applied from the buccal arm on the appliance to the bracket via elastic.

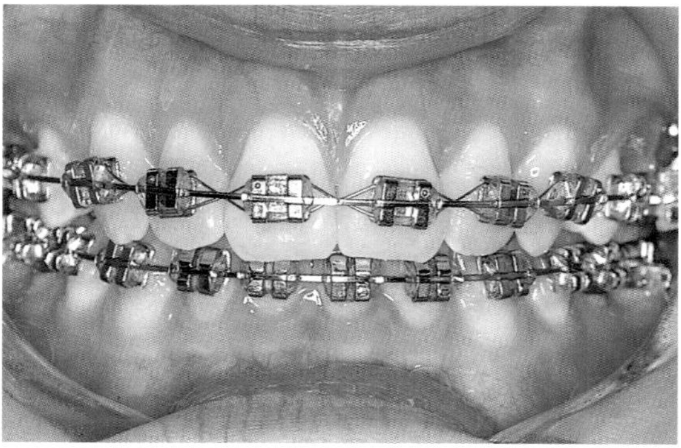

**Fig. 83** Pre-adjusted edgewise appliance – Andrews' prescriptions.

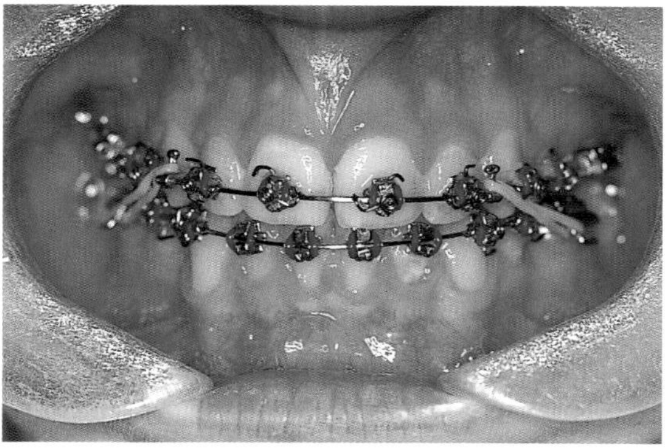

**Fig. 84** Tip-edge appliance.

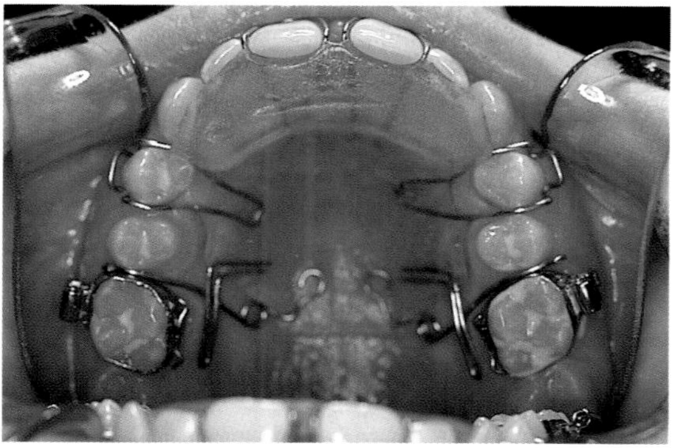

**Fig. 85** URA with bands on $\underline{6}$s for extraoral traction.

# 17 / Functional appliances

*Definition*

An appliance using, removing or modifying the forces generated by the orofacial musculature, tooth eruption and dentofacial growth.

*Types of functional appliances*

These are usually given the name of their originator, e.g. Harvold, Bionator (after Balters; Fig. 86), Frankel (Fig. 87). Most are 'one-piece' appliances, except twin-block (Fig. 88); the Herbst appliance is a fixed functional appliance. Twin-block may also be cemented. Headgear can be added to some functional appliances (e.g. twin-block) when maximal anteroposterior and vertical maxillary restraint is desirable and/or if FMPA is increased.

*Mechanism of action*

The mechanism is incompletely understood. Forces are developed by posturing the mandible (downward and forward in Class II cases; downward and backward in Class III cases). Scope for the former is much greater than for the latter, therefore appliances are used almost exclusively in Class II cases to apply intermaxillary traction. These appliances apply or eliminate forces produced by facial and masticatory muscles, and harness those occurring through natural growth processes. They are only effective in growing children, preferably just pre-pubertal. Appliance design influences the specific force system generated.

*Practical management*

To be effective, the appliance should be worn for at least 14 hours per day. Review 1–2 weeks after fitting and then at 6–8 week intervals. Record the overjet with the mandible in maximum retrusion at each review visit. Slight occlusal over-correction is advisable, and then the appliance should be worn as a retainer at night until growth has reduced to adult levels or until the second phase of treatment starts. If there is no progress in the first 6 months, stop treatment and reassess.

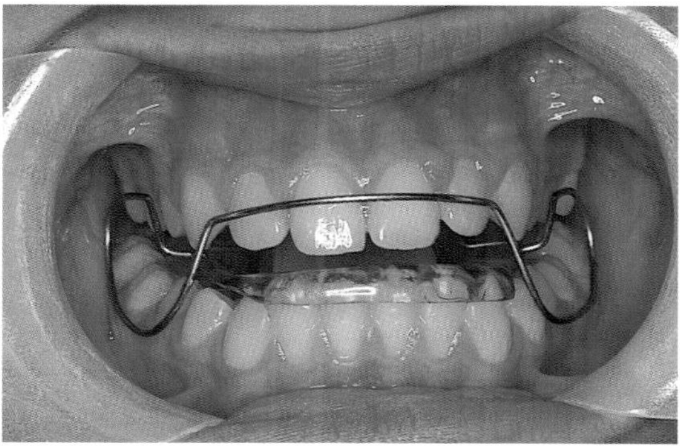

**Fig. 86** Bionator appliance.

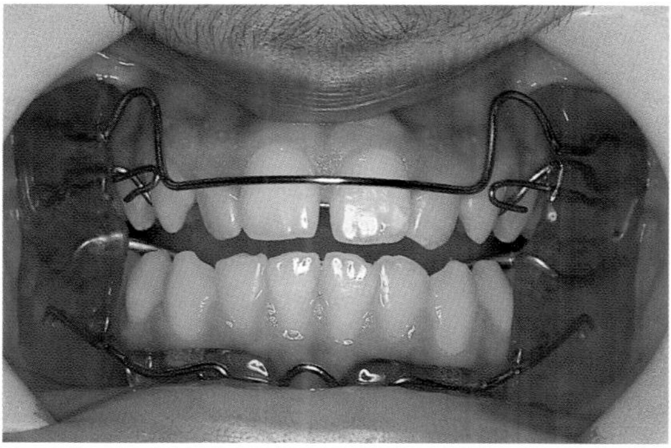

**Fig. 87** Frankel II appliance.

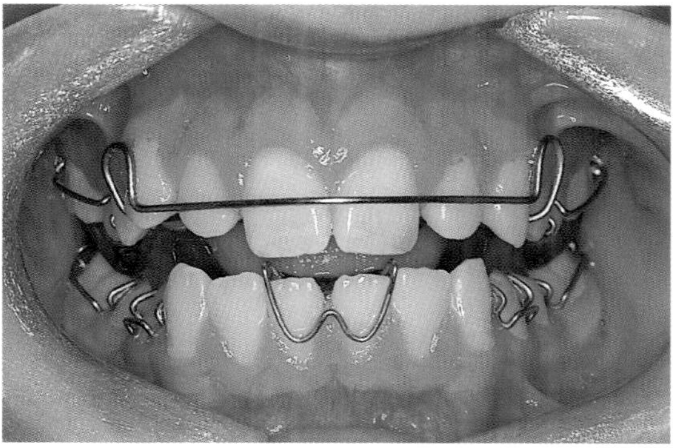

**Fig. 88** Twin-block appliance.

## Indications

As the sole means of Class II correction in a growing child if the following conditions are met: mild skeletal Class II due to mandibular retrusion; average/reduced FMPA; uncrowded arches; upright or slightly retroclined lower incisors (Fig. 89a, b). (Functional appliances have limited use for Class III or anterior open bite correction (pp. 49, 55).

May also be used for the preliminary phase of treatment in mixed dentition in severe Class II malocclusion to aid occlusal correction prior to fixed appliances and possibly extractions.

## Effects (Figs 89a–d)

When used for correction of Class II with deep overbite:

### Skeletal

Enhancement of mandibular growth by movement of mandibular condyle out of the fossa promoting condylar cartilage growth and anterior migration of glenoid fossa (effect very variable); inhibition of forward maxillary growth; lower facial height increase (Figs 89a–d).

Overall growth is modified, the total amount of mandibular growth is unaffected, but growth expression is altered.

### Dental

Retroclination of upper incisors/proclination of lower incisors; inhibition of lower incisor eruption; promotion of mesial and upward eruption of lower posterior teeth; prevention of eruption and mesial movement of upper posterior teeth. Arch expansion in some cases.

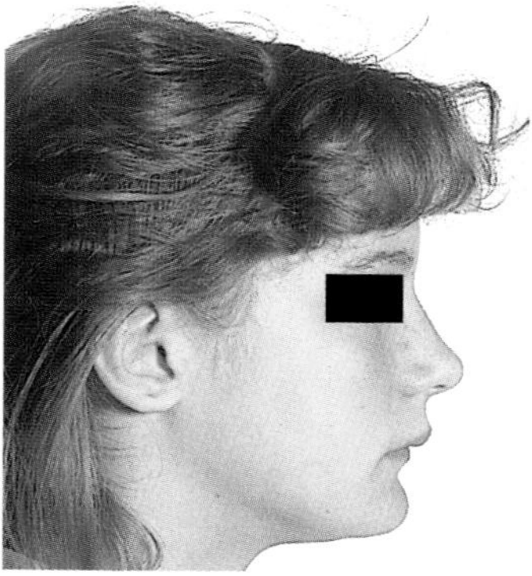

**Fig. 89a** Pre-treatment: Class II skeletal pattern.

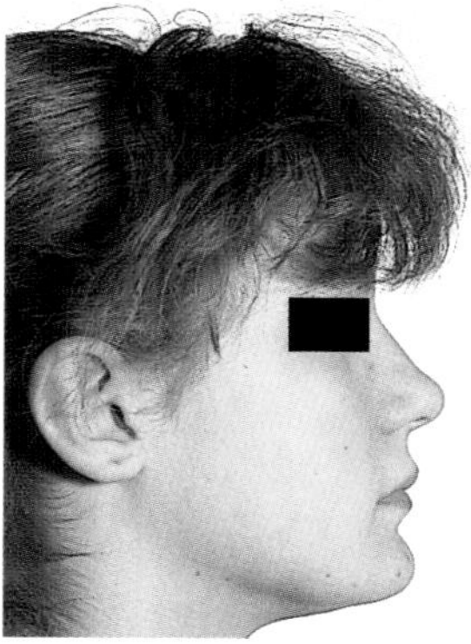

**Fig. 89b** Post-treatment: Profile.

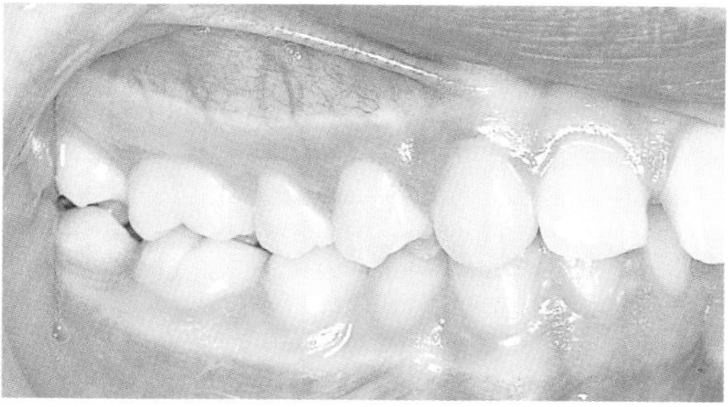

**Fig. 89c** Pre-treatment occlusion.

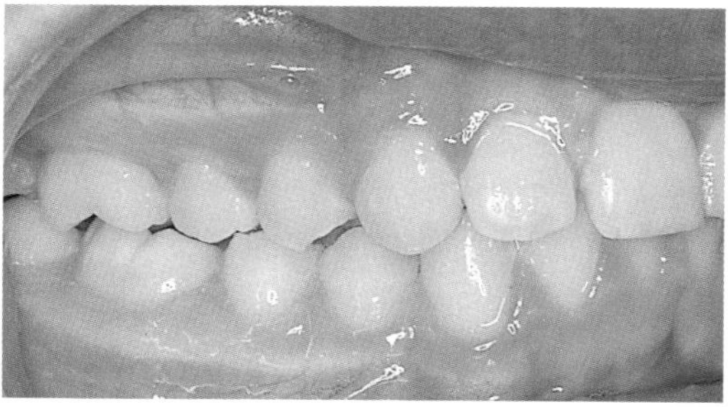

**Fig. 89d** Post-treatment occlusion (note the slight overcorrection).

# 18 / Adult orthodontics

## Special considerations

- Adults are usually highly motivated but also have high expectations.
- There is a greater likelihood of systemic disease (e.g. diabetes), and adults are more prone to periodontal disease.
- There may be a compromised dentition, such as periodontal disease, tooth loss, extensive restorative treatment (Fig. 90) with perhaps retained roots, periapical pathology or root resorption. Multidisciplinary input is often necessary to achieve the best result.
- Lack of growth means that skeletal discrepancies other than mild ones are often best dealt with by an orthodontic/surgical approach rather than by camouflage. Where camouflage is considered, overbite reduction by incisor intrusion rather than by molar extrusion is necessary.
- Anchorage planning in adults is more demanding than in adolescents due to previous tooth loss and/or reduced bony support (Fig. 91). Headgear is not realistic – use palatal/lingual arches.
- Reduced cell population, and often reduced vascularity of alveolar bone, mean slower initial tooth movement but otherwise movement is as efficient as in adolescents. Retention is often lengthy as there is slower tissue remodelling and it must be permanent if there is reduced periodontal support.
- Lighter forces are required in reduced periodontium.
- There is less adaptation to disruption in occlusion, so stable functional occlusion post-treatment must be ensured.
- Aesthetic brackets are often required to improve the appearance of the appliance (Fig. 92).

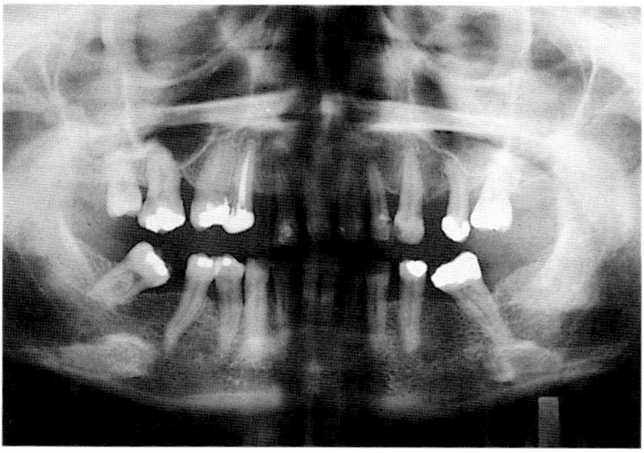

**Fig. 90** Compromised adult dentition.

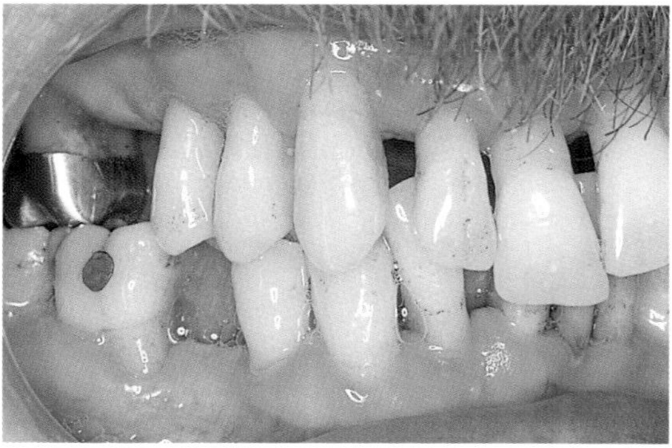

**Fig. 91** Tooth loss and reduced periodontal support.

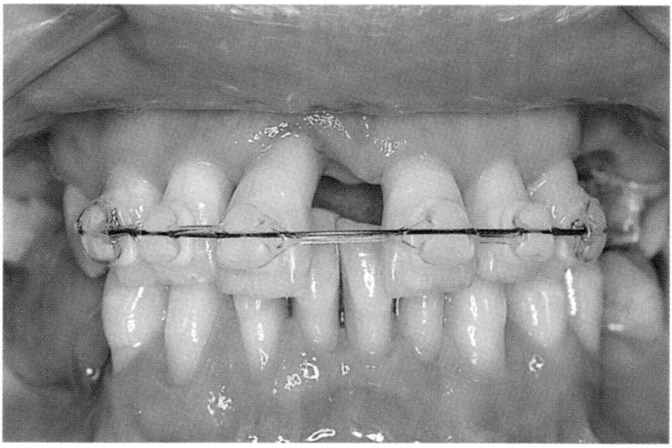

**Fig. 92** Tooth-coloured brackets.

## Treatment

### Adjunctive

Aim to correct one aspect of malocclusion to improve dental health or function. Typically treatment is of $\leq$ 6 months duration and integrated with periodontal or advanced restorative procedures (e.g. crossbite correction, alignment of drifting incisors (Fig. 93a, b), uprighting of teeth prior to bridgework, extrusion of teeth with subgingival fracture).

### Comprehensive

Aim to achieve an optimal aesthetic and functional occlusal result. If there is mild skeletal discrepancy, camouflage by dentoalveolar movement is possible with fixed appliances. The principles are similar for major malocclusion types but overbite reduction is by intrusion rather than by molar extrusion (Fig. 94). If there is a more marked skeletal discrepancy, a combined surgical/ orthodontic approach is required. Comprehensive treatment can still be undertaken where significant loss of periodontal support is present, provided that disease has been controlled before treatment and there is regular periodontal recall during treatment.

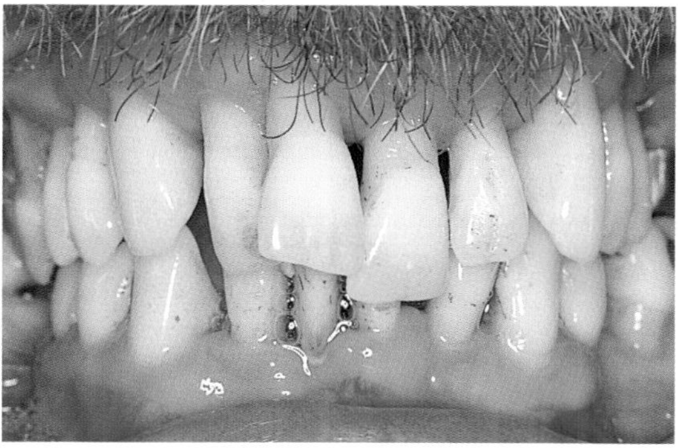

**Fig. 93a** Pre-treatment with drifting incisors.

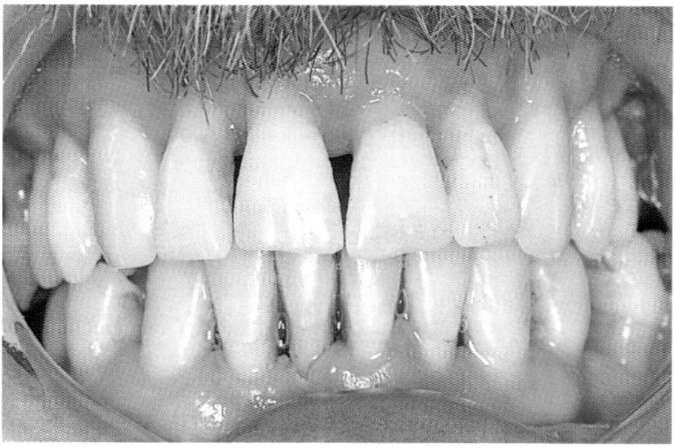

**Fig. 93b** Following fixed appliance alignment of labial segments.

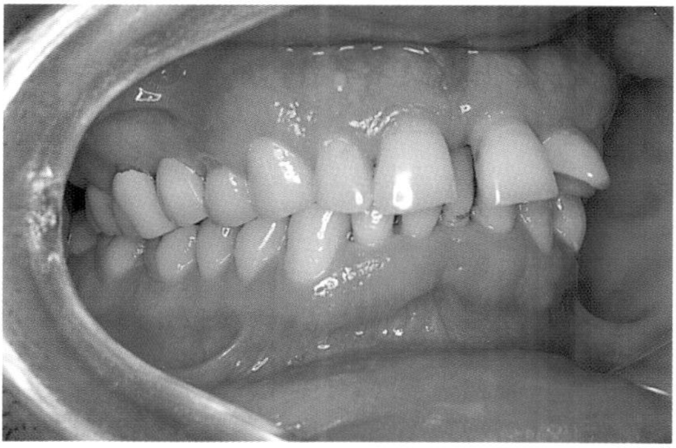

**Fig. 94** Adult patient where incisor intrusion is required for overbite reduction.

# 19 / Surgical orthodontic treatment

*Definition*

Correction of dentofacial deformity through a combined surgical and orthodontic approach.

*Timing of treatment*

Usually carried out when growth is essentially complete, but intervention may be earlier if the temporomandibular joint (TMJ) is ankylosed, or there is severe psychological distress due to deformity.

*Indications*

Moderate to severe anteroposterior (Fig. 95), vertical (Fig. 96), lateral (Fig. 97) skeletal discrepancies as well as craniofacial anomalies, including cleft lip and palate.

*Planning surgical–orthodontic treatment*

- A team approach is essential. Treatment often requires the input of a plastic surgeon, a restorative specialist, a clinical psychologist and a speech therapist in addition to the orthodontist and oral and maxillofacial surgeon.
- Ascertain the patient's complaint – dental and/or facial appearance, masticatory function, speech, or a combination of these? Psychological assessment indicated?
- Obtain a detailed medical and dental history, and perform a thorough analysis of facial form and profile, including temporomandibular joint.
- Obtain facial and dental photographs, panoramic and lateral cephalometric films and dental casts. Posteroanterior (PA) cephalometric film is required if there is facial asymmetry. CT scans are needed in complex syndromes.

*Record analysis and planning*

- Superimpose a standard skull template matched for age and racial group (e.g. Bolton standard) on the patient's cephalometric tracing (Fig. 98) to indicate areas of discrepancy. Templates, however, are a composite of males and females.
- Plan surgical changes using enlarged full face and profile photographs matched for size to the cephalometric tracing, or by a computer programme or video imaging system.
- Simulate surgical movements on a duplicate set of study models. Mount on semi-adjustable articulator if bimaxillary procedure is planned.

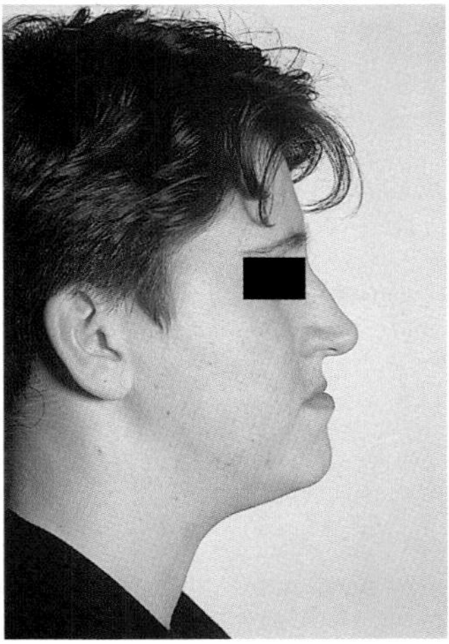

**Fig. 95** Moderately severe Class III skeletal discrepancy.

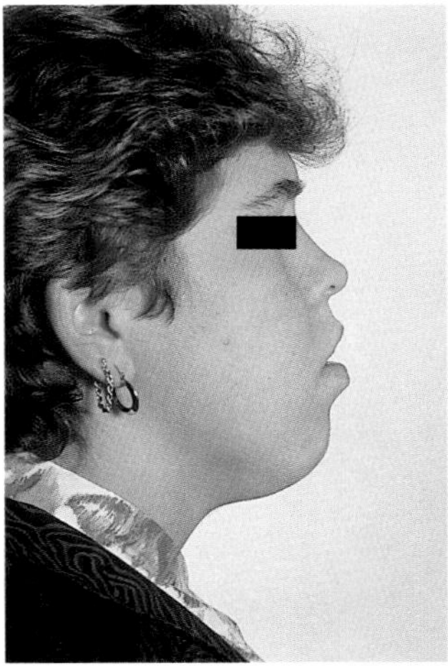

**Fig. 96** Markedly increased lower anterior face height.

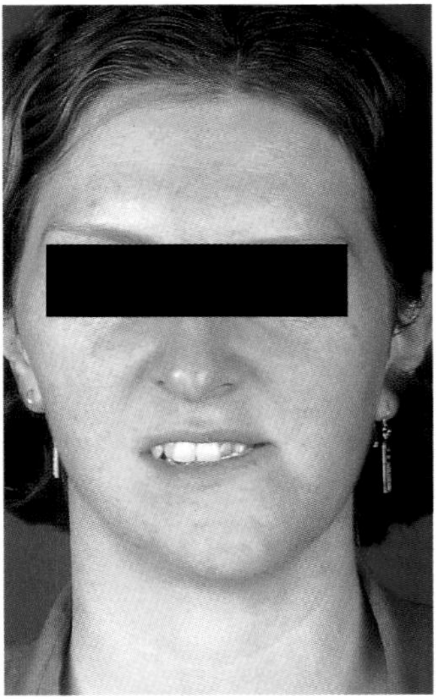

**Fig. 97** Severe facial asymmetry.

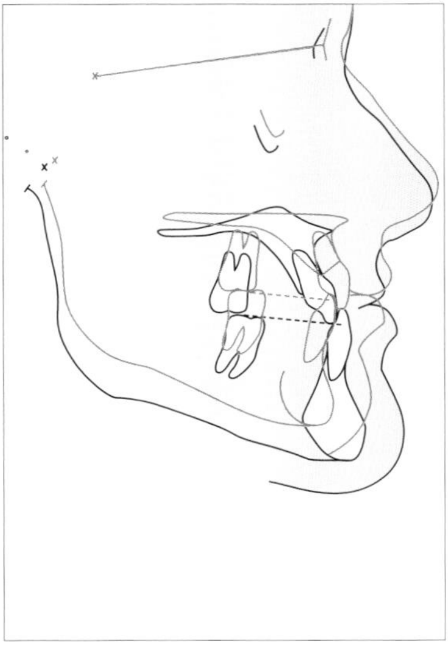

**Fig. 98** Bolton standard (blue) superimposed on computer-generated tracing.

## Orthodontic management

*Pre-surgical orthodontics*

Usually decompensate for any dentoalveolar compensation so that true jaw discrepancy is revealed (Fig. 99a, c). Align and coordinate arches or arch segments and establish the vertical and anteroposterior position of the incisors so that jaws can be positioned in the desired location without interference from tooth positions. Place rigid rectangular stabilising archwires with ball hooks pre-surgically.

*Post-surgical orthodontics*

Intermaxillary traction on round lighter wires to finalise occlusal result. Retention regime is usually as follows fixed appliance therapy. Surgical follow-up for a minimum of 2 years.

*Stability*

This is enhanced when surgical movement is modest and does not induce soft tissue tension (Fig. 99b, d).

## Surgical procedures

*Maxilla*

*Le Fort I osteotomy.* This is the most common procedure. It allows repositioning of the maxilla superiorly, inferiorly or anteriorly.

*Le Fort II osteotomy.* This allows correction of marked maxillary retrognathism and nasal retrusion.

*Le Fort III osteotomy.* Used to correct Crouzon's syndrome. It may be combined with a Le Fort I osteotomy.

*Segmental procedures.* These include Wassmund for premaxillary prominence; they are now used rarely since there is a risk of root damage from interdental cuts.

*Mandible*

*Sagittal split osteotomy.* Inferior dental nerve damage is common.

*Vertical subsigmoid osteotomy.* Used to correct mandibular prognathism.

*Body osteotomy.* Useful if existing space or space created by extraction orthodontically. Valuable if there is mandibular prognathism and asymmetry.

*Sub-apical osteotomy.* Usually of the anterior dentoalveolar segment only, but may involve the entire arch. Loss of pulpal vitality is possible.

*Genioplasty.* Allows chin repositioning.

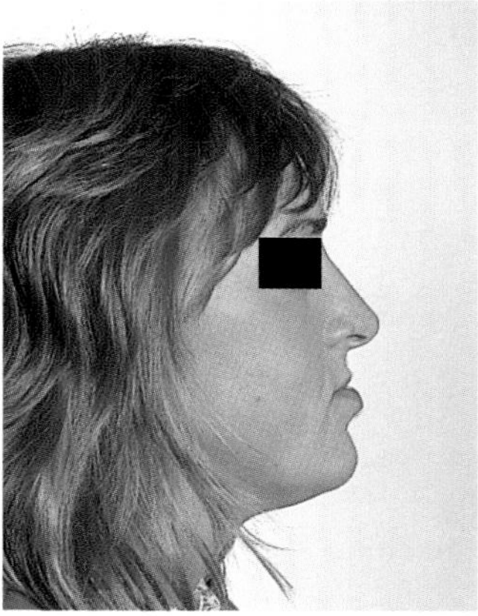

**Fig. 99a** Post-decompensation: profile.

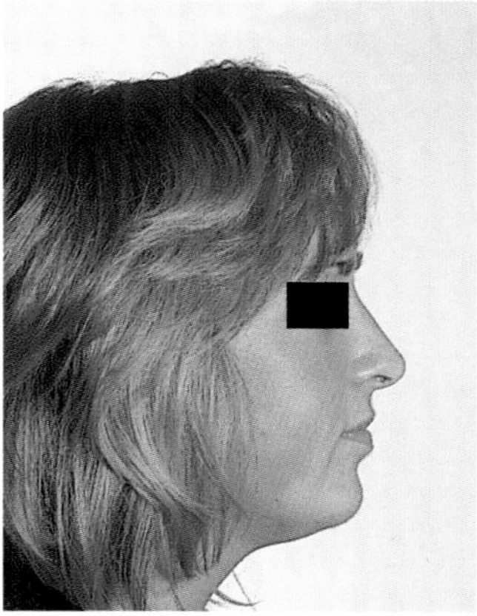

**Fig. 99b** 1 year post-bimaxillary osteotomy: profile.

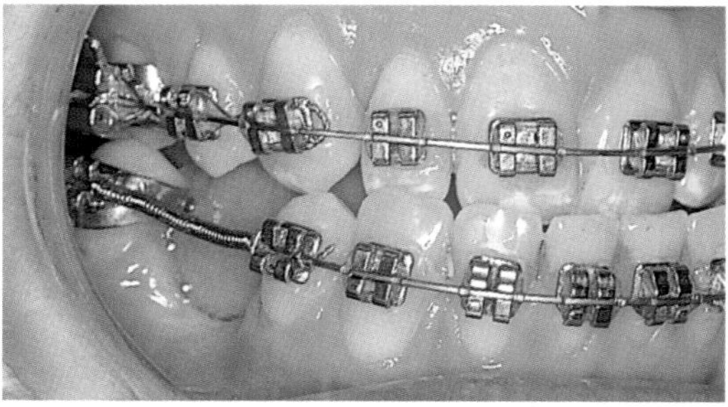

**Fig. 99c** Occlusion (post-decompensation).

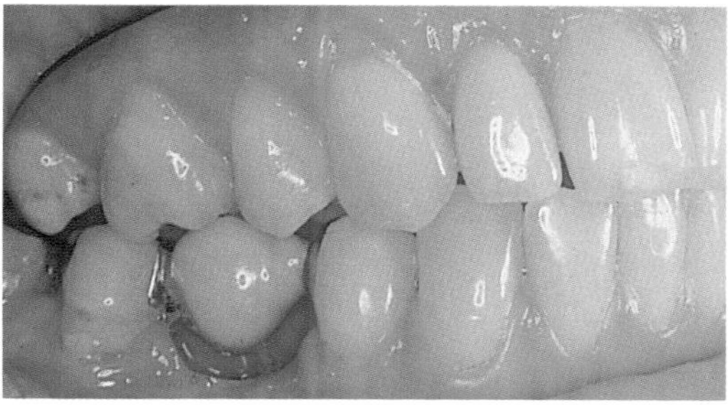

**Fig. 99d** Occlusion (1 year post-surgery).

# 20 / Cleft lip and palate CL(P)

*Prevalence*

In Caucasians, CL(P) occurs in 1 in 750 live births; CP in 1 in 2000 live births. CL(P) is more common in males; CP is more common in females.

*Aetiology*

Aetiology is incompletely understood. There is a family history in 40% of CL(P) and in 20% of CP cases. Genetic predisposition may possibly be triggered by environmental factors.

*Classification*

Primary palate (lip and alveolus to the incisive foramen) and/or secondary palate (hard palate from incisive foramen back and soft palate), unilateral or bilateral, complete or incomplete (Figs 100, 101). Also submucous cleft.

## Common clinical features

*Skeletal*

Patients show a tendency to retrognathic maxilla and mandible; reduced upper and increased lower face height with excess freeway space. Class III skeletal relationship is common.

*Dental and occlusal*

On the cleft side, $\underline{2}$ is either absent, of abnormal size and/or shape, hypoplastic or as two conical teeth on either side of the cleft; a supernumerary or supplemental tooth may exist on either side of the cleft; $\underline{1}$ is often rotated and tilted towards the cleft and may be hypoplastic, particularly in bilateral cases; eruption is delayed. Tooth size elsewhere in the mouth tends to be smaller. Class III incisor relationship is common with crossbite of one or both buccal segments and occasionally a lateral open bite (Fig. 102).

*Growth*

Post-surgical scarring in patients with CL + P restricts midfacial growth.

*Hearing and speech*

Hearing difficulties are common in patients with CP. Palatal fistulae and adverse palatopharyngeal function impair speech.

*Other anomalies*

Cardiac and digital anomalies are present in about a fifth of those with clefts, and are most common in those with CP only.

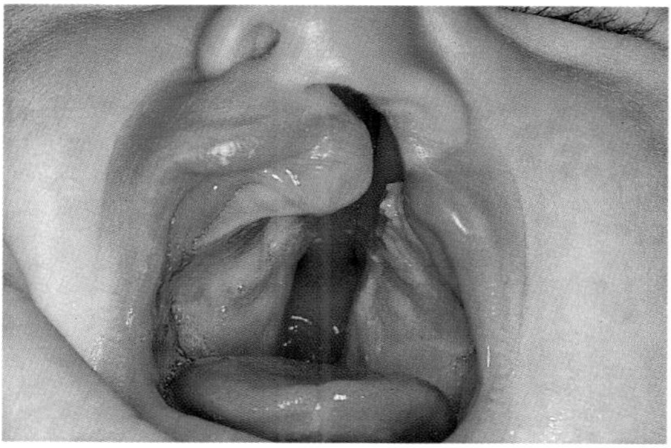

**Fig. 100** Left complete unilateral cleft lip and palate.

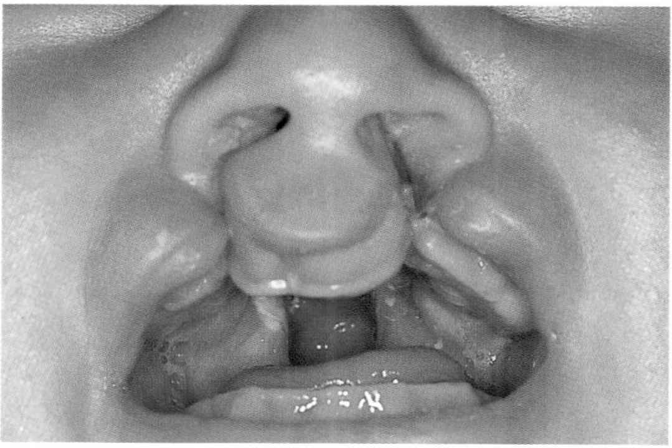

**Fig. 101** Bilateral complete cleft lip and palate.

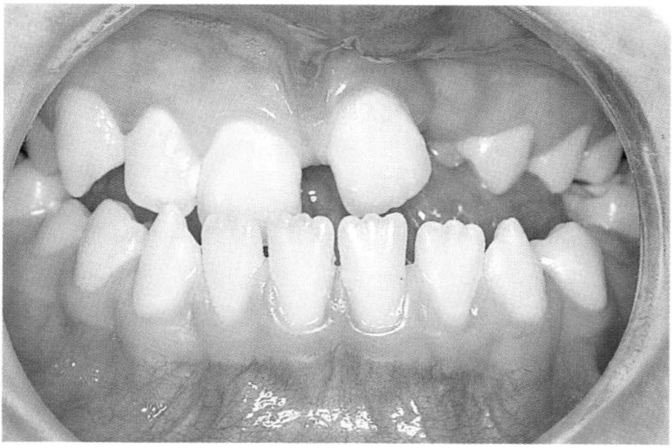

**Fig. 102** Occlusion in a patient with left unilateral cleft lip and palate.

## Management of care

This is best coordinated in a specialised centre by a team comprising orthodontist, speech therapist, health visitor, plastic, ENT and maxillofacial surgeons. Dental care should be monitored regularly by a general dental practitioner.

**Neonatal period to 18 months**
Parental counselling and reassurance by the orthodontist; feeding instruction; advice and support from a specialised health visitor. Pre-surgical orthopaedics may be needed to reposition displaced cleft segments. Lip closure is usually carried out at 3 months (usually Millard technique), with bilateral lip repair in either one or two stages. Palate repair is usually at 9–12 months (usually von Langenbeck procedure).

**Primary dentition**
Preventive advice; regular speech and hearing assessment; speech therapy as required. Possibly pharynoglasty and/or lip revision at 4–5 years.

**Mixed/permanent dentition**
Correct incisor crossbite in early mixed dentition or postpone until preparation for alveolar bone grafting (8–11 years). Usually align incisors and expand upper arch prior to bone grafting. Graft restores arch integrity (Fig. 103a, b), allows eruption of $\underline{3}$, space closure, supports alar base and aids closure of oronasal fistulae. Once $\underline{3}$ erupts, correct the centreline and move buccal segments forward so $\underline{3}$ replaces missing or diminutive $\underline{2}$. Consider relief of crowding in the non-cleft quadrant and in the lower arch. Delay lower arch extractions if orthognathic surgery is planned.

**In late teenage years**
If there is gross midface retrusion (Fig. 104), Le Fort I or II advancement is likely with possible mandibular setback and/or genioplasty. Consider rhinoplasty later.

**Retention**
Bonded permanent retention in the upper arch in all cases.

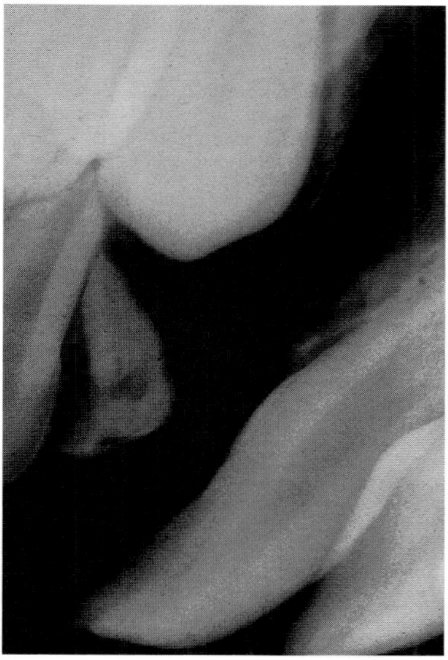

**Fig. 103a** Pre-alveolar bone grafting.

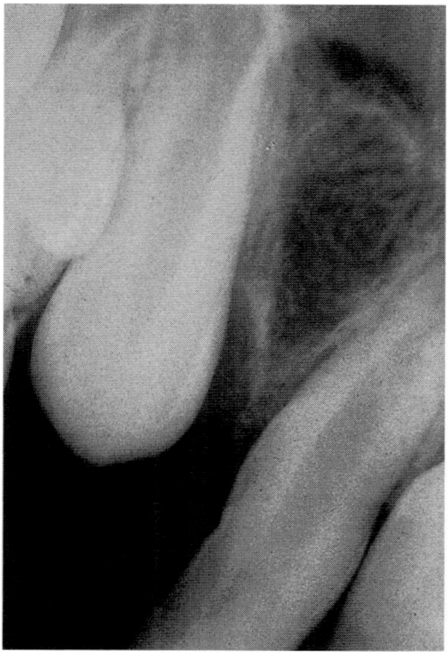

**Fig. 103b** Post-alveolar bone grafting. Note 3| erupting through the graft.

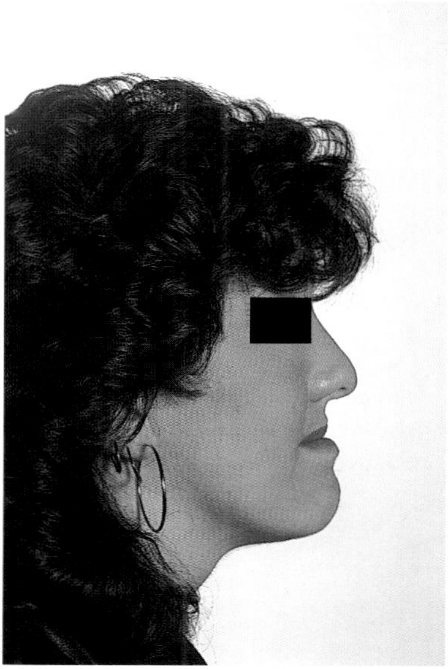

**Fig. 104** Midface retrusion in a patient with repaired cleft palate.

# 21 / Tooth eruption

*Primary teeth* erupt at the following times: incisors 6–9 months; first molars 12–14 months; canines 16–18 months; second molars 20–24 months.

*Permanent teeth* erupt at the following times: incisors 6–9 years; first molars 6–7 years; lower canines 9–10 years; first premolars 10–11 years; second premolars 11–12 years; upper canines 11–12 years; second molars 11–13 years; third molars 17–21 years.

## Natal/neonatal teeth

*Definition*

Natal (present at birth). Neonatal (erupt within 28 days of birth).

*Incidence*

1 in 700 to 1 in 6000 births.

*Clinical features*

They are usually lower incisors (Fig. 105) of the normal dentition (only 10% are supernumeraries). They may cause tongue trauma, nipple trauma (if the child is breast fed), or be a danger to the airway if they are very mobile.

*Management*

Retain if possible. Extract for any of above reasons.

## Eruption cyst

*Aetiology and pathology*

A type of dentigerous cyst.

*Clinical features*

Smooth, rounded swelling with a bluish appearance, sited on the alveolar ridge where a tooth will erupt (Fig. 106).

They usually, but not always, affect primary teeth and permanent molars (i.e. teeth with no predecessors).

*Management*

Reassurance. This is a self-limiting condition. Rarely, analgesia and antibiotics are required.

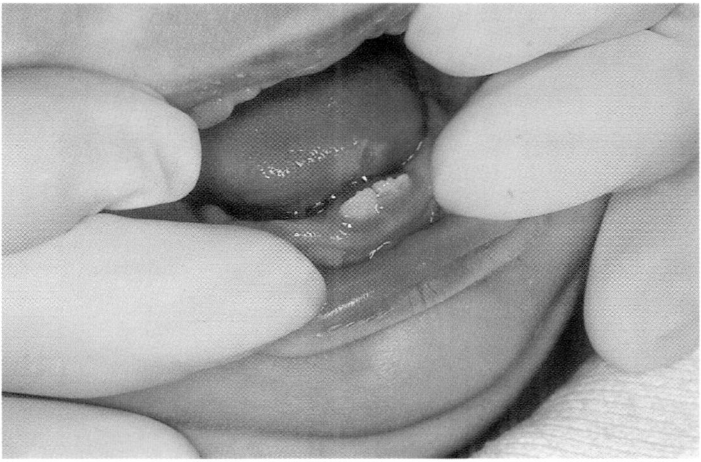

**Fig. 105** Neonatal teeth.

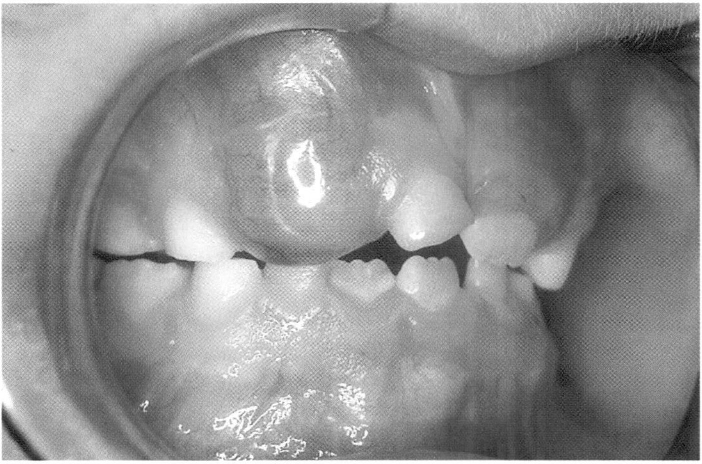

**Fig. 106** Eruption cyst over an upper permanent incisor.

# 22 / Nursing and rampant caries

## Nursing caries

*Definition*

Anterior caries in the pre-school child. 'Nursing caries' is now the preferred term. Previous terms included bottle caries and baby bottle tooth decay (Figs 107, 108, 109).

*Aetiology and pathology*

Frequent or prolonged consumption of fluids containing fermentable carbohydrates (or non-milk extrinsic (NME) sugars) from a bottle; feeder cup or on-demand nightly breast-feeding after 15 months of age.

*Clinical features*

Lower incisors are rarely affected as they are protected during suckling by the tongue and directly bathed in secretions from the sublingual and submandibular glands.

Progression of decay is rapid, commencing on the labial surfaces and quickly encircling the teeth.

Teeth are affected in the order of eruption. Classically affected teeth are the upper incisors, canines and first molars, and lower first molars.

*Management*

- Dietary advice – eradicate frequent on-demand liquids at night.
- Water only should be available at night.
- Discing interdentally to make self-cleansing together with regular fluoride application or build-up with strip crowns.

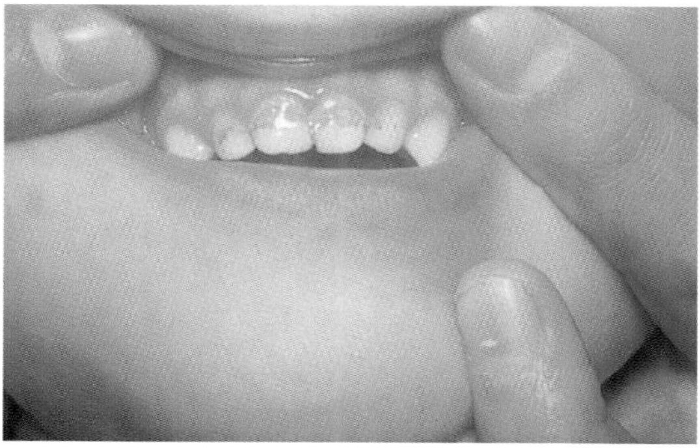

**Fig. 107** Early nursing caries.

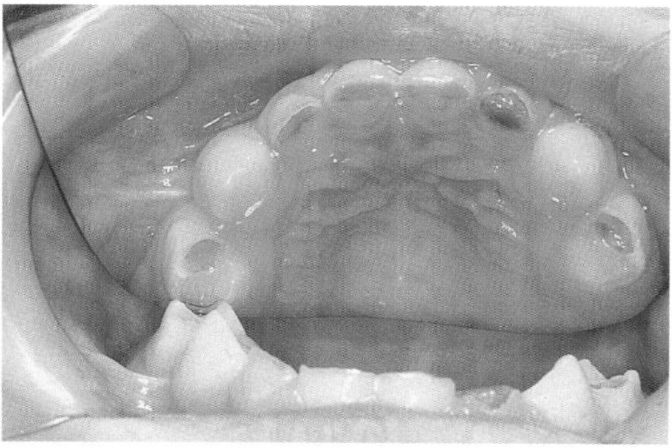

**Fig. 108** Nursing caries of the upper incisors and first primary molars.

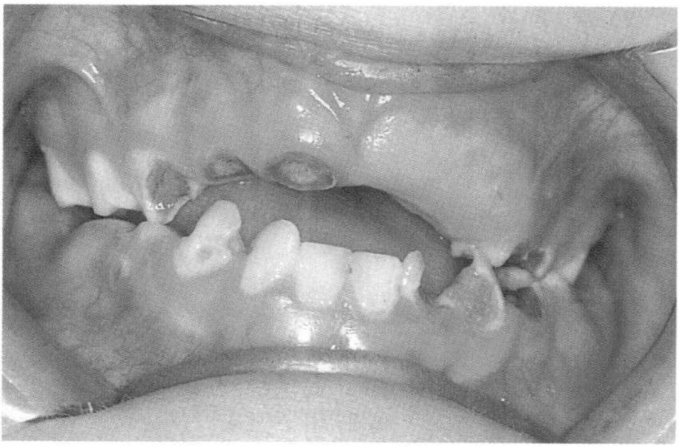

**Fig. 109** Severe nursing caries.

## Rampant caries

*Definition*

Caries progresses from a nursing caries pattern to involve lower anterior primary teeth and second primary molars.

*Aetiology and pathology*

Frequent consumption of liquids and foods containing non-milk extrinsic (NME) sugars.

*Clinical features*

Can involve any tooth, primary and permanent, as they erupt (Figs 110, 111, 112).

*Management*

*Prevention.* 3 day dietary analysis. Optimal systemic and topical fluoride. Toothbrush instruction. Fissure sealant placement on first permanent molars as they erupt.

*Restoration/extraction.*

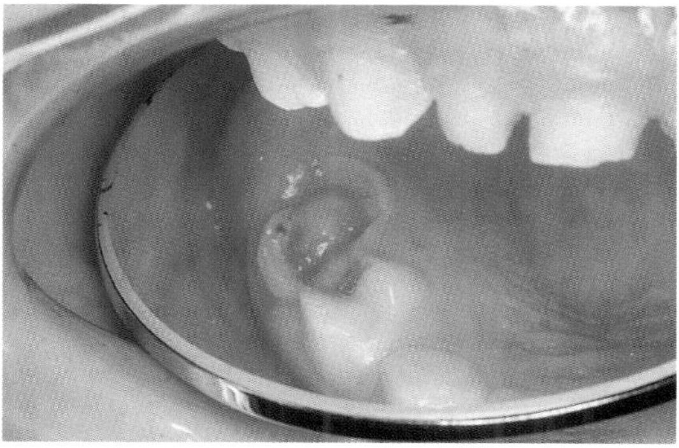

**Fig. 110** Rampant caries with a pulp polyp of the upper second primary molar.

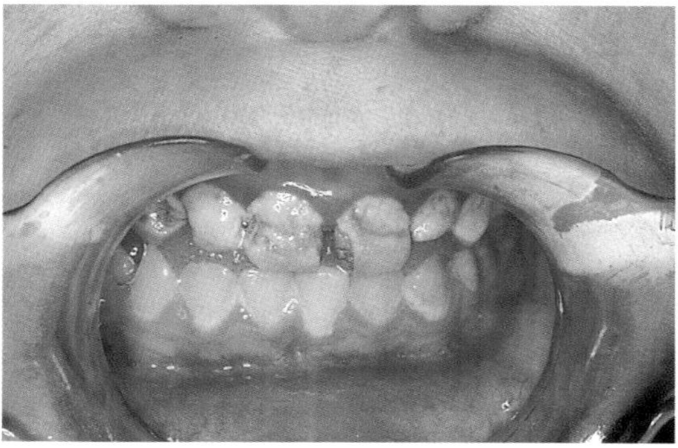

**Fig. 111** Rampant caries with poor oral hygiene.

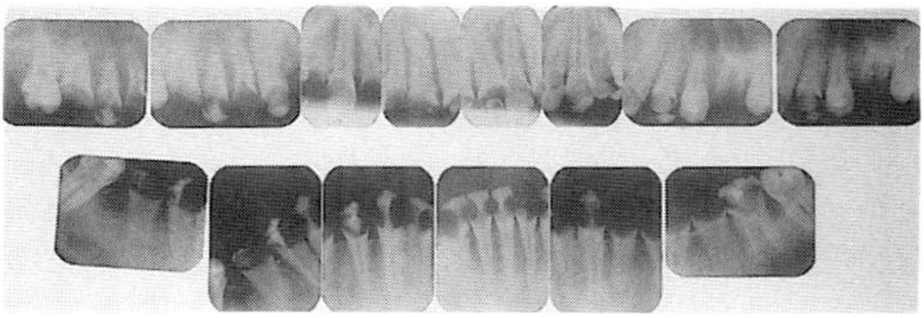

**Fig. 112** Rampant caries due to polo mint addiction.

# 23 / Tooth discoloration

## Extrinsic

*Aetiology*

*Beverages/food.*

*Poor oral hygiene (chromogenic bacteria)*: green/orange stain.

*Drugs*: iron supplements – black; minocycline – black; chlorhexidine – brown/black; rifabutin – red.

*Clinical features*

*Poor oral hygiene*: gingivally (Fig. 113).

*Beverages/food*: affects all surfaces but mainly gingivally (Fig. 114).

*Drugs*: affects all surfaces but mainly gingivally.

*Management*

- Reassurance.
- If due to beverages/food/drugs, it can be removed by prophylaxis.
- Poor oral hygiene requires tooth brush instruction with the use of disclosing tablets/solution (Fig. 115).

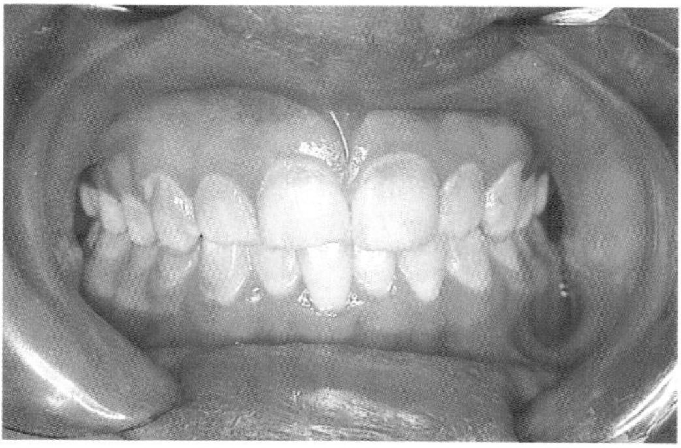

**Fig. 113** Chromogenic extrinsic stain due to poor oral hygiene.

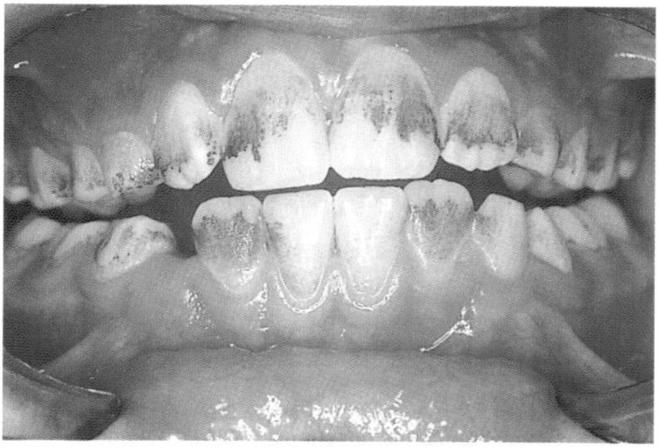

**Fig. 114** Black extrinsic stain secondary to beverages/food.

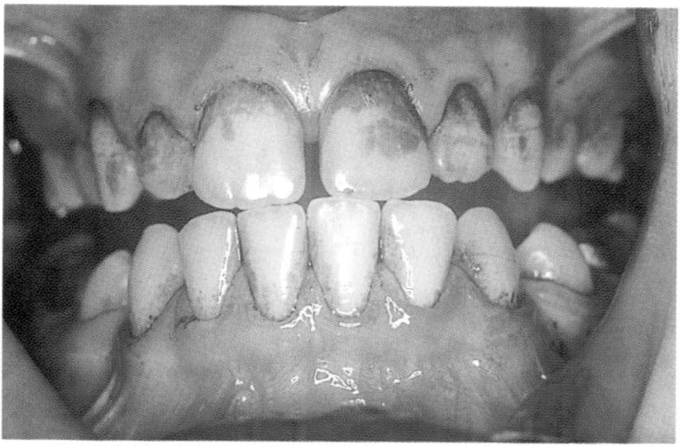

**Fig. 115** Disclosing solution identifying plaque deposits.

## Intrinsic

*Aetiology: enamel*

*Local.*

- Caries
- Idiopathic
- Injury/infection of primary predecessor
- Internal resorption.

*Systemic.*

- Amelogenesis imperfecta
- Drugs (e.g. tetracycline) (Fig. 116)
- Fluorosis
- Idiopathic
- Illness during tooth formation.

*Aetiology: dentine*

*Local.*

- Caries
- Internal resorption
- Metallic restorative materials
- Necrotic pulp tissue (Fig. 117)
- Root canal filling materials.

*Systemic.*

- Bilirubin (liver disease) (Fig. 118)
- Congenital porphyria
- Dentinogenesis imperfecta
- Drugs (e.g. tetracycline) (Fig. 116).

*Clinical features and management*

Specific to each cause.

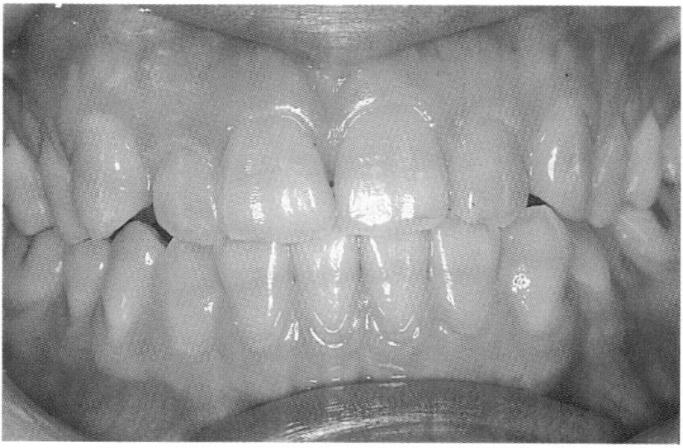

**Fig. 116** Tetracycline staining.

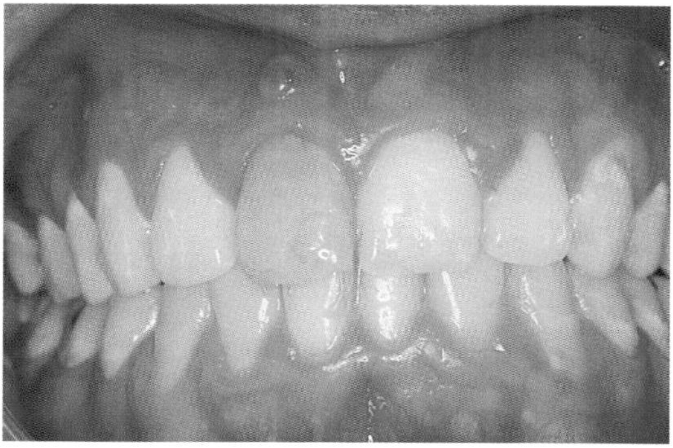

**Fig. 117** Non-vital tooth discoloration.

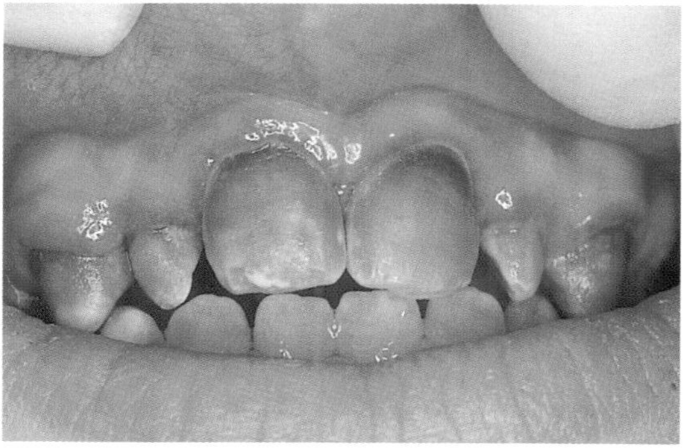

**Fig. 118** Green staining of haemoglobin breakdown products in a liver transplant patient (prepared for veneers in upper arch).

# 24 / Enamel hypoplasia and fluorosis

## Enamel hypoplasia

*Aetiology*

Tooth development can be disturbed by constitutional disturbances. Maternal illness during pregnancy can affect all primary teeth and first permanent molar teeth (Figs 119, 120). Childhood febrile illness or gastroenteritis can affect the adult dentition (Fig. 121). These disturbances produce a linear pattern of hypoplasia corresponding to the site of amelogenesis at the time ('chronological' hypoplasia).

Infection or trauma to a primary tooth may cause hypoplasia of the underlying permanent successor.

*Clinical features*

Hypoplasia related to medical, dental and trauma history.

*Management*

Restoration of original morphology with appropriate materials.

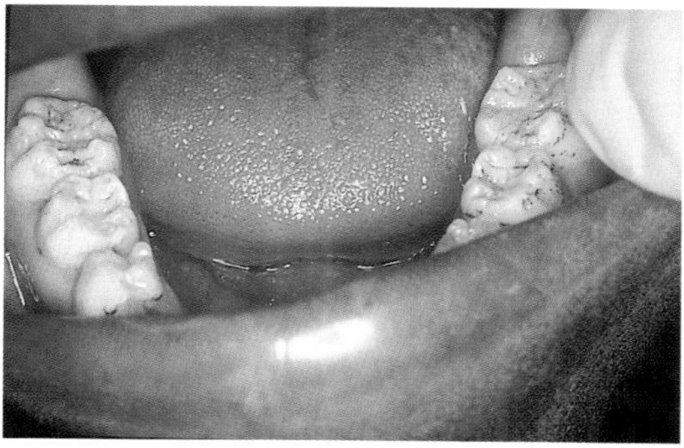

Fig. 119 Enamel hypoplasia of primary and permanent molars.

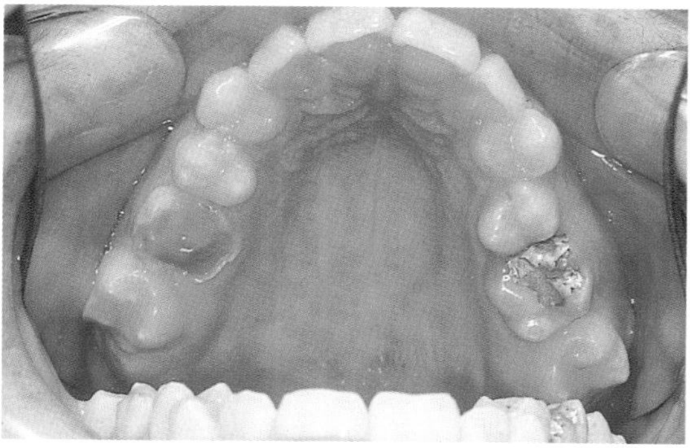

Fig. 120 Enamel hypoplasia of permanent first molars.

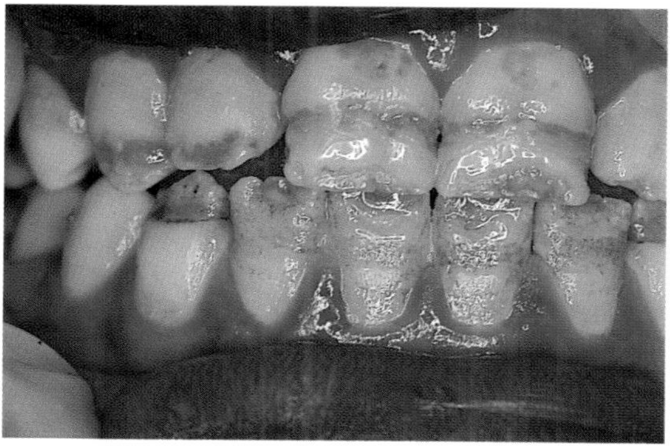

Fig. 121 Enamel hypoplasia of permanent anteriors.

## Fluorosis

*Aetiology and pathology*

Amelogenesis can be disturbed by excessive chronic ingestion of fluoride either from naturally occuring sources in drinking water or from overdosage by fluoride supplements and toothpastes, or by a combination of the two.

It can occur in the primary dentition but is largely confined to the permanent dentition. 20–24 months of age is a particularly vulnerable time for upper permanent central incisors.

It commonly affects the outer enamel layers.

*Clinical features*

May vary from diffuse white opaque lines to scattered white flecking, or a more opaque and confluent dense white chalky mottling that may contain brown discoloration (Figs 122, 123), or all the above with pitting hypoplasia.

*Differential diagnosis*

Other causes of intrinsic discoloration.

*Management*

Acid pumice microabrasion. Composite veneers.

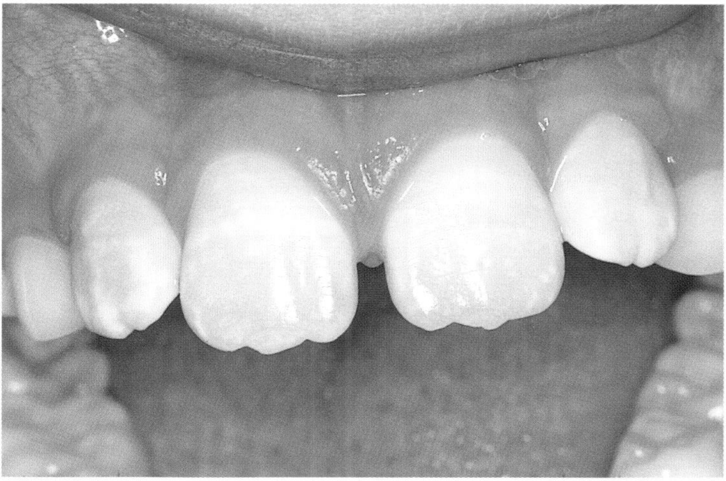

**Fig. 122** Diffuse fluorosis.

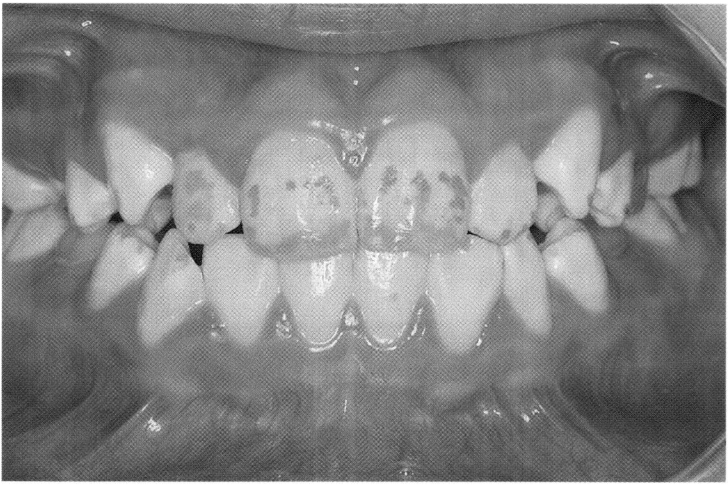

**Fig. 123** Dense fluorosis.

# 25 / Inherited anomalies

## Amelogenesis imperfecta

*Aetiology and pathology*

Genetic with different 'modes' of inheritance as well as a wide variety of presentations. Incidence is 1 in 10000.

*Clinical features*

There are three main types of enamel anomaly:

*Hypoplastic.* There is a deficiency of matrix but normal calcification of matrix which is present. The enamel is pitted and irregular and retains extrinsic stain (Fig. 124).

*Hypocalcified.* The enamel matrix is normal but there is inadequate calcification. The enamel may be normal in the gingival third of the tooth. Affected enamel is often opaque and retains stain. It is soft and easily lost (Fig. 125).

*Hypomature.* The enamel matrix is normal but there is little maturation or calcification of the enamel and the enamel is soft and porous (Fig. 126).

*Differential diagnosis*

Other causes of intrinsic discoloration.

*Management*

Complex treatment plan consisting of: stabilisation/protection of the posterior occlusion with onlays or preformed crowns, followed by improvement of anterior aesthetics with composite veneers.

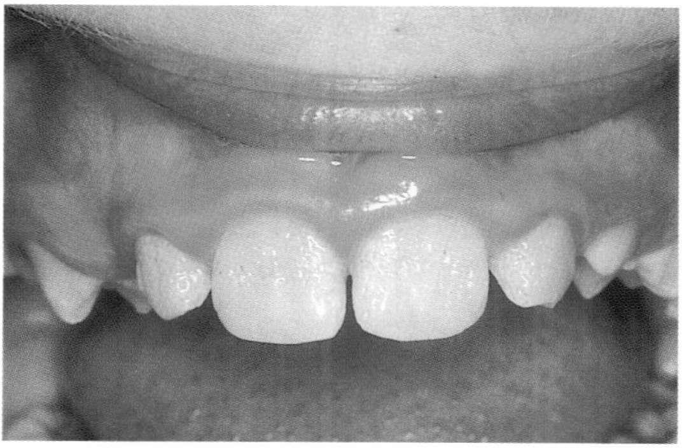

**Fig. 124** Hypoplastic amelogenesis imperfecta.

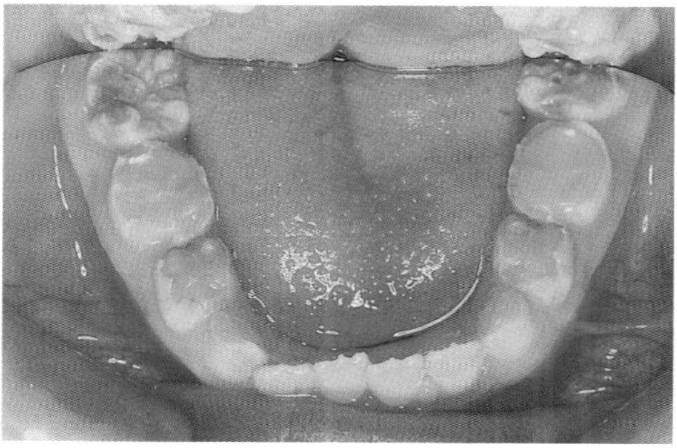

**Fig. 125** Hypocalcified amelogenesis imperfecta.

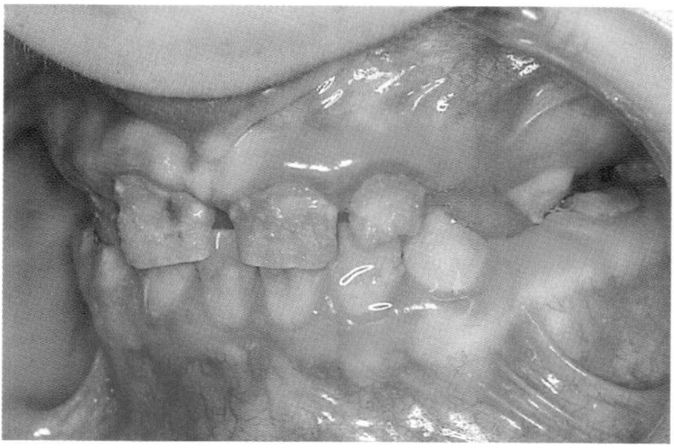

**Fig. 126** Hypomature amelogenesis imperfecta.

## Dentinogenesis imperfecta

*Aetiology and pathology*

Autosomal dominant inheritance. Incidence is 1 in 8000.

*Clinical features*

Dentine is abnormal in structure and is translucent.

Three main types exist:

- Type I (associated with osteogenesis imperfecta)
- Type II (hereditary opalescent dentine)
- Type III (brandywine type).

Types I and II are similar: primary teeth are more severely affected than permanent teeth. In the permanent dentition, teeth which develop first may be more severely affected than those which develop later.

The teeth are translucent and vary in colour from grey to blue or brown (Figs. 127, 128). Enamel is poorly adherent to abnormal dentine and easily chips and wears. Crowns are bulbous with pronounced cervical constriction. Radiographically there are shortened roots, progressive pulp chamber and canal obliteration, and spontaneous periapical abscess formation (Fig. 129).

*Differential diagnosis*

Other causes of intrinsic discoloration.

*Management*

Complex treatment plan consisting of: stabilisation/protection of the posterior occlusion with onlays or preformed crowns followed by improvement of anterior aesthetics with composite veneers.

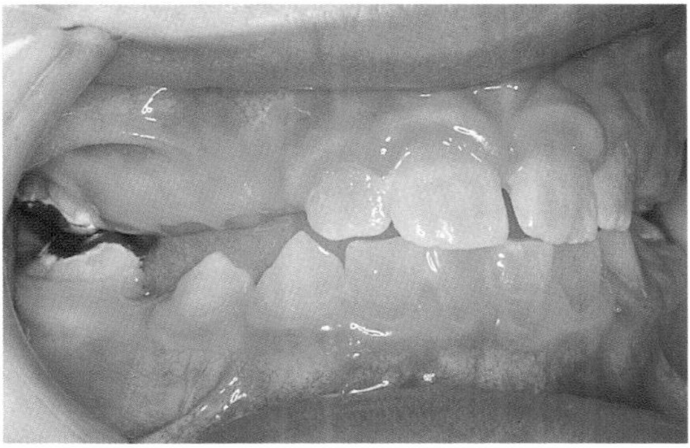

**Fig. 127** Dentinogenesis imperfecta. Onlays on first permanent molars.

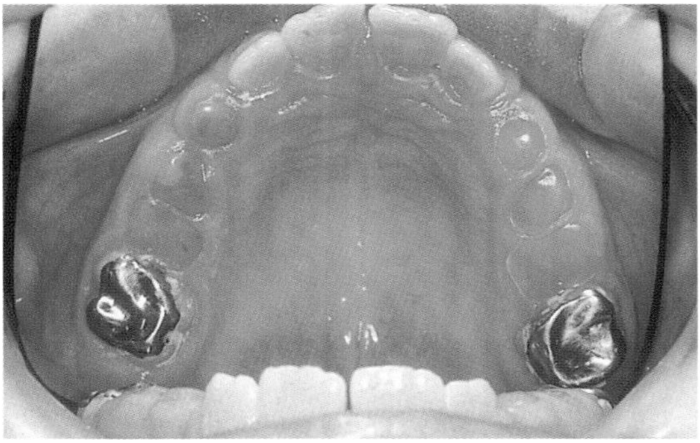

**Fig. 128** Dentinogenesis imperfecta. Onlays on first permanent molars.

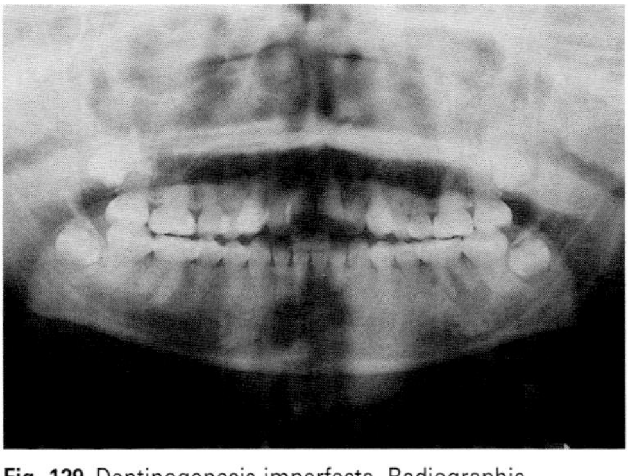

**Fig. 129** Dentinogenesis imperfecta. Radiographic appearance.

## Hyperdontia

*Definition*

Additional teeth can either resemble the normal dentition (supplemental) (Fig. 130) or be a simple conical or tubercular shape (supernumerary). Midline supernumeraries are also called mesiodens and may be inverted (Fig. 131). Unerupted supernumeraries often impede normal tooth eruption (see p. 19).

*Incidence and aetiology*

1.5–3.5% of the population. Multifactorial genetic inheritance.

*Clinical features*

Associated with syndromes: cleidocranial dysplasia; Gardner's syndrome; Hallermann–Streiff syndrome; cleft lip and palate.

*Management*

Normal extraction or surgical removal. For orthodontic management see page 19.

## Hypodontia

*Definition*

Absence of one or more teeth.

*Incidence and aetiology*

3.5–6.5% of the population (not counting third molars).

Multifactorial genetic inheritance, cytotoxic drugs, radiotherapy.

*Clinical features*

Hypodontia of genetic origin usually affects the last tooth in a series: lateral incisors (Fig. 132); second premolars; third molars. Microdontia (small teeth) is an expression of hypodontia.

Associated with syndromes: Albright's osteodystrophy; hypothyroidism; Down syndrome; ectodermal dysplasia; Goltz syndrome; Hallermann–Streiff syndrome; orofaciodigital syndrome; cleft lip and palate.

*Management*

Joint orthodontic, prosthodontic, oral surgery and paediatric dentistry treatment planning. For orthodontic management see p. 21.

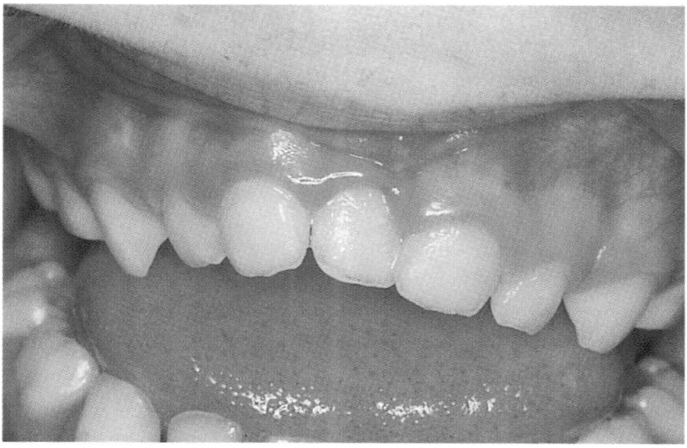

**Fig. 130** Supplemental upper primary incisor.

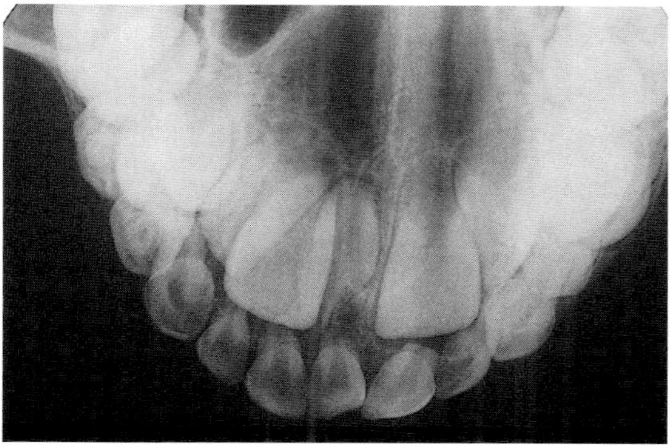

**Fig. 131** Radiograph of Fig. 130. A supernumerary permanent incisor is present between developing central incisors.

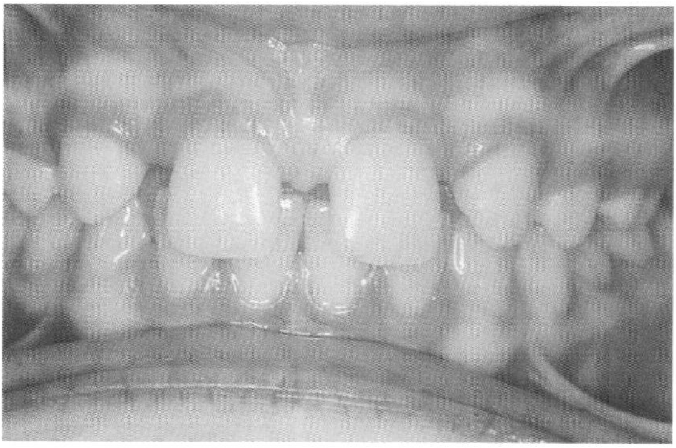

**Fig. 132** Absent upper lateral incisors.

## Talon cusp

*Definition*

Prominent additional cusp.

*Clinical features*

Commonly on the buccal surface of primary first molars, the palatal surface of primary second molars, and palatal surfaces of permanent incisor teeth (Fig. 133).

*Management*

Maxillary permanent incisor 'talon' cusps often cause malocclusion and may require removal and elective root treatment once the root is fully formed.

## Odontomes

*Definition*

Non-neoplastic, developmental anomalies or malformations derived from dental formative tissues.

*Complex odontome* is an irregular mass of recognisable enamel, dentine and pulp (Fig. 134).

*Compound odontome* is a collection of numerous discrete tooth-like structures with enamel dentine and pulp arranged as in a normal tooth.

*Dilated odontome* (dens in dente; dens invaginatus) is an invagination of enamel and dentine to form a pouch of enamel (Fig. 135).

*Clinical features*

Compound and complex odontomes obstruct normal tooth eruption. Dilated odontomes are prone to caries and pulpal infection.

*Management*

Surgical removal of compound and complex odontomes. Dilated odontomes may be root-treated as long as the pouch of enamel is coronal, and can be removed competely. Otherwise usually extraction is required.

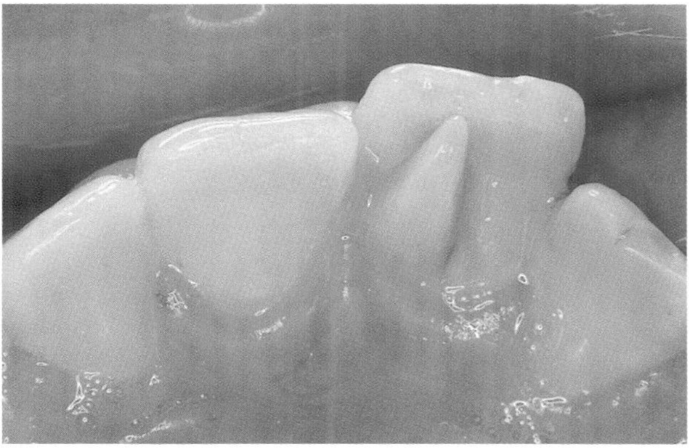

**Fig. 133** Talon cusp.

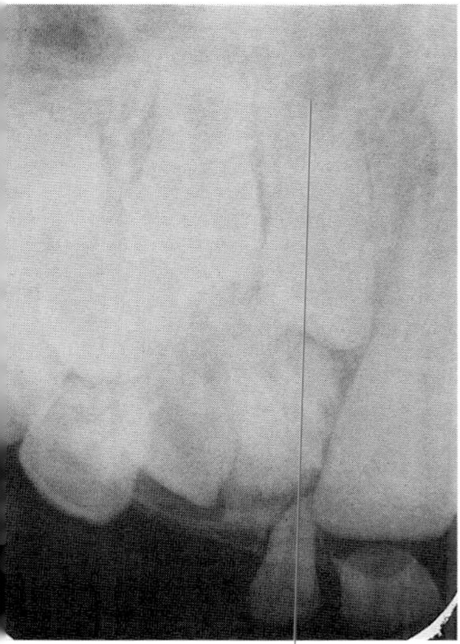

**ig. 134** Odontome obstructing upper right
ateral. The upper right primary canine is
lso impacted.

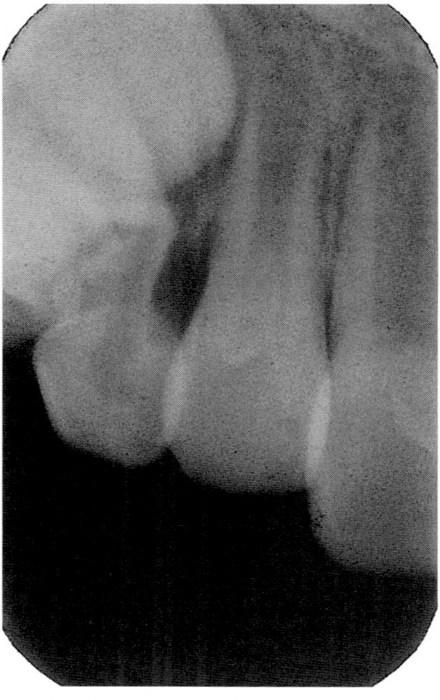

**Fig. 135** Dens in dente of upper lateral incisor.

# 27 / Autotransplantation

*Definition*

Transplantation of a tooth in the upper or lower arch to a prepared socket in the same mouth (Fig. 136).

*Incidence*

Increasingly common and successful treatment of trauma cases where an incisor has been lost or in hypodontia cases where there may be crowding in other quadrants.

*Clinical features*

Lower first and second premolars are the easiest teeth to transplant.

*Management*

Combined treatment planning with orthodontics, oral surgery and paediatric dentistry.

Ideally, root formation of the transplanted tooth should be two-thirds complete, so that revascularisation may occur.

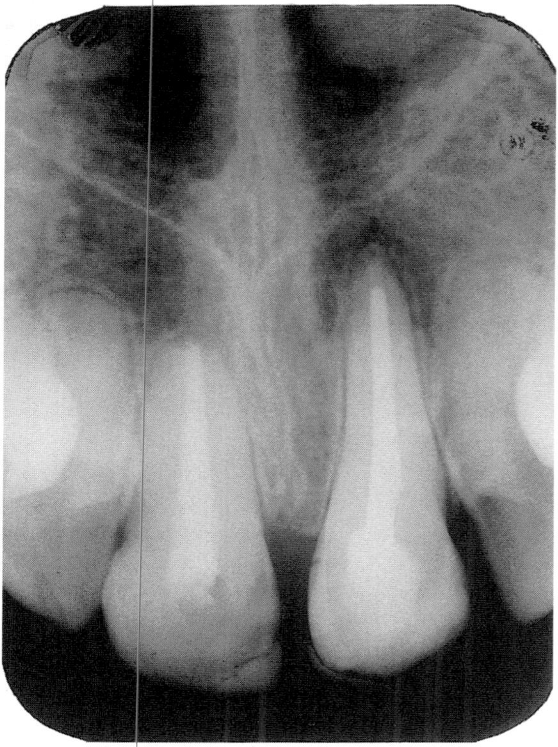

**Fig. 136** Autotransplanted canine in upper central region.

# 28 / Tooth surface loss

*Definition and classification*

Non-carious loss of tooth tissue. There are three main types:

*Attrition.* Wear of a tooth as a result of tooth-to-tooth contact.

*Abrasion.* Physical wear by something other than tooth-to-tooth.

*Erosion.* Wear by a chemical process not involving bacteria (Figs 137, 138, 139).

This is the predominant form of tooth wear in paediatric dentistry.

## Erosion

*Incidence*

- 52% of 5-year-olds have palatal erosion on upper primary incisors.
- 27% of 15-year-olds have palatal wear on upper permanent incisors.

*Aetiology*

*Dietary.*
- Citrus fruits
- Fruit juices
- Carbonated drinks
- Vinegar and pickles
- Yoghurt
- Vitamin C tablets.

*Gastric regurgitation.*
- Gastro-oesophageal reflux
- Oesophageal strictures
- Chronic respiratory disease
- Overfeeding
- Mental disability
- Feeding problems.

*Management*

- Dietary modification.
- Composite/metal veneers or onlays.

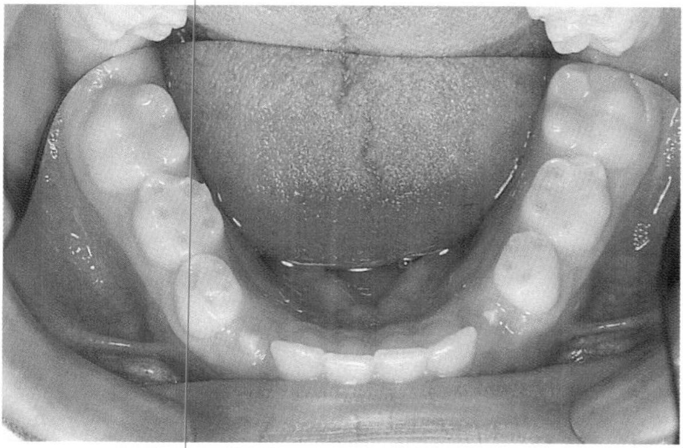

**Fig. 137** Early erosion of primary molars.

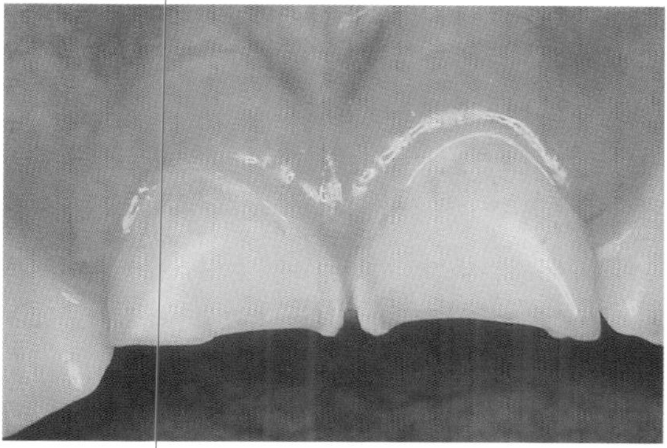

**Fig. 138** Labial and incisal erosion of permanent incisors.

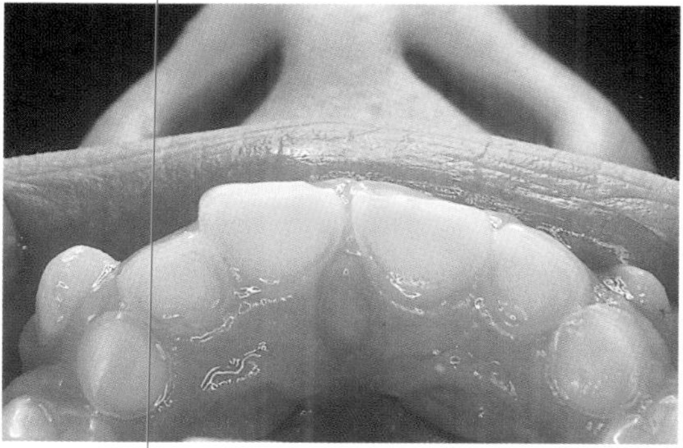

**Fig. 139** Palatal erosion of permanent incisors.

# 29 / Primary tooth trauma

*Incidence* 16–40% of children by 5 years of age. Twice as many boys as girls.

*Classification* World Health Organization (WHO) classification.

*Aetiology* Majority of injuries at 2–4 years of age are due to falls during normal walking or playing.

*Clinical features* Commonest injuries are displacements (Fig. 140) rather than crown fractures. This is due to the elasticity of young bone.

*Management* If cooperation allows, enamel dentine fractures can be restored and non-vital primary incisors can be root-filled with zinc oxide (Fig. 141).

Displacement injuries may be treated conservatively in the absence of pain, occlusal disturbances or excessive motility if the root of the primary tooth is displaced away from the permanent tooth germ.

If root displacement is towards the permanent tooth germ or any of the above criteria are present, then extraction is necessary.

*Complications*

- Primary tooth pulp death.
- Damage to underlying permanent successor tooth.

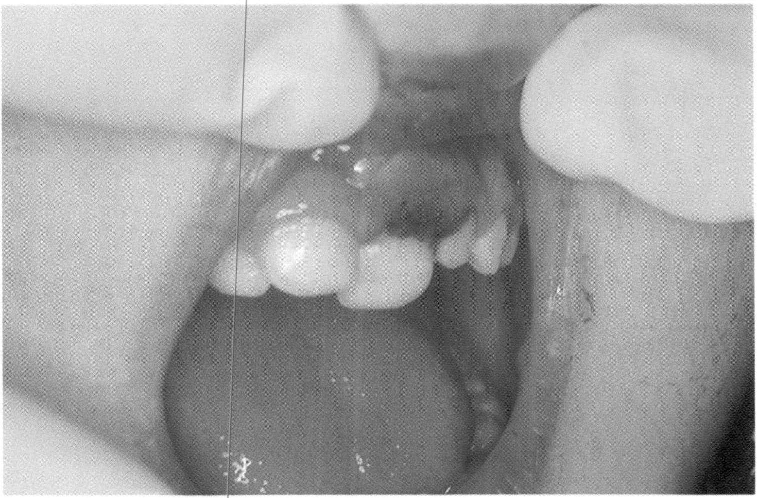

Fig. 140 Luxation of primary incisors.

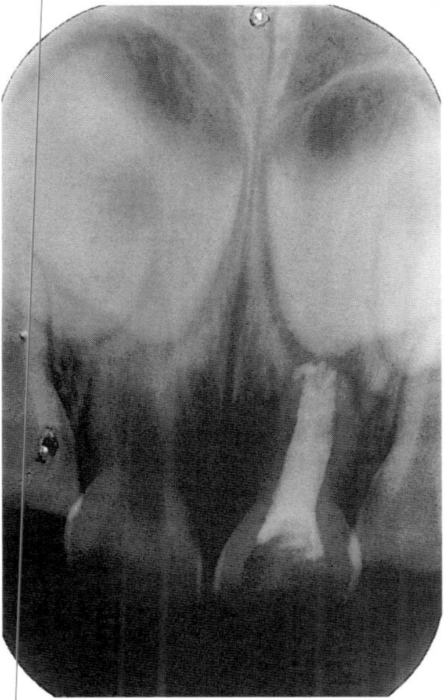

Fig. 141 Root-filled primary incisor.

## Damage to permanent teeth after primary tooth trauma

*Incidence*

Up to 60% of primary tooth injuries.

*Classification*

- Hypoplasia of enamel (Fig. 142)
- Dilaceration of crown/crown root/root (Fig. 143)
- Odontoma-like malformation
- Root duplication
- Partial or complete arrest of root formation
- Sequestration of permanent germs
- Disturbance in eruption.

*Aetiology*

Disturbance of amelogenesis or root formation by either direct contact of the primary tooth or oedema surrounding the primary tooth root (Fig. 144).

*Clinical features*

Specific to the classification.

*Management*

Wide spectrum involving orthodontics, oral surgery and paediatric dentistry, depending on the anomaly.

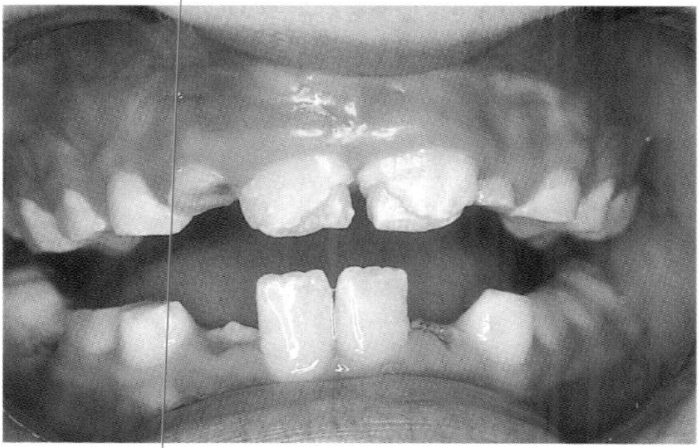

Fig. 142 Permanent incisor enamel hypoplasia.

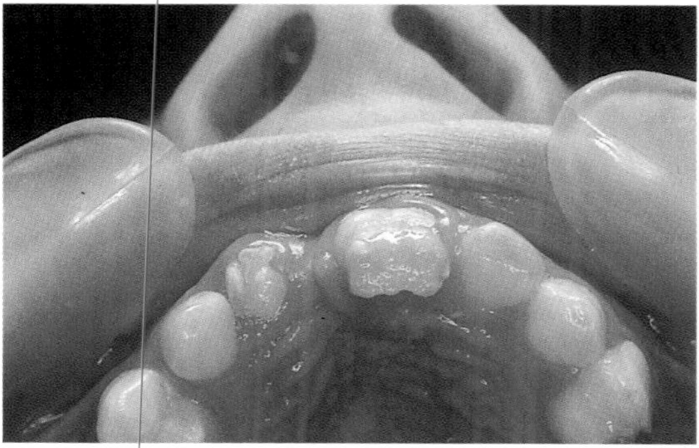

Fig. 143 Dilaceration of permanent central incisor crown.

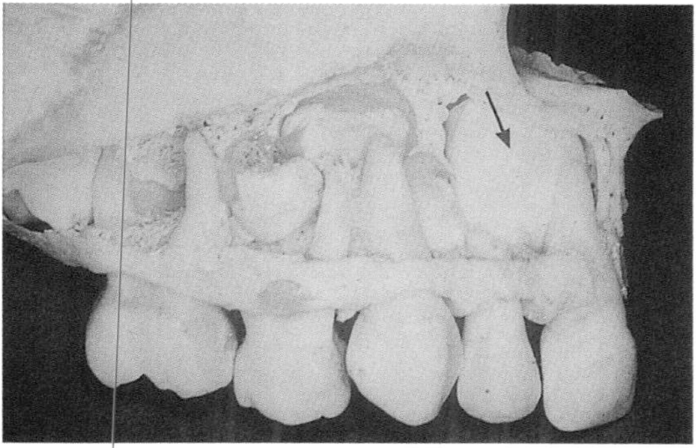

Fig. 144 Anatomy of developing dentition.

# 30 / Permanent tooth trauma I

| | |
|---|---|
| *Incidence* | 4–33% of children by 12 years of age. Twice as many boys as girls. |
| *Classification* | World Health Organization (WHO) classification. |
| *Aetiology* | Majority of injuries occur at 7–10 years of age due to falls during normal play. |
| *Clinical features* | Commonest injuries are uncomplicated (enamel dentine) crown fractures (Fig. 145). |
| *Management* | Appropriate management demands accurate diagnosis and will include any of the following:<br>• Protection of exposed dentine.<br>• Pulp treatment which will differ depending on apical maturity.<br>• Monitoring of apical development (Figs 146, 147).<br>• Reduction and splinting of displacement and avulsion injuries.<br>• Treatment of soft tissue or intra-bony infection.<br>• Anterior aesthetic considerations. |
| *Complications* | • Pulp death.<br>• Root resorption. |

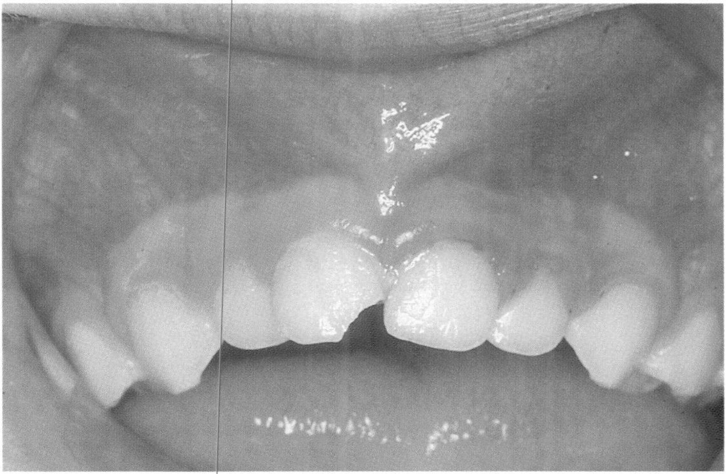

**Fig. 145** Enamel dentine fracture.

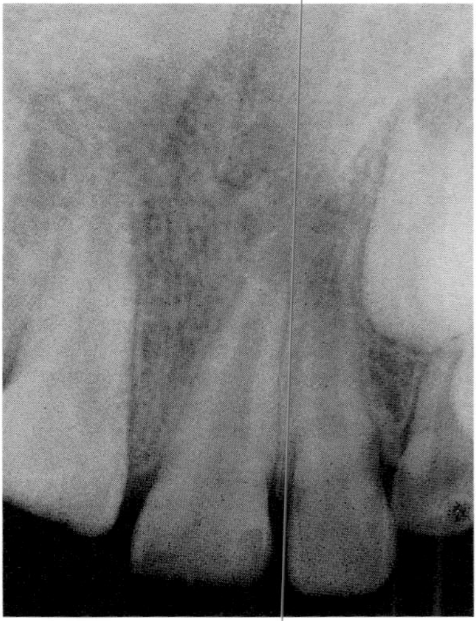

**Fig. 146** Enamel dentine fracture; immature apex, left central incisor.

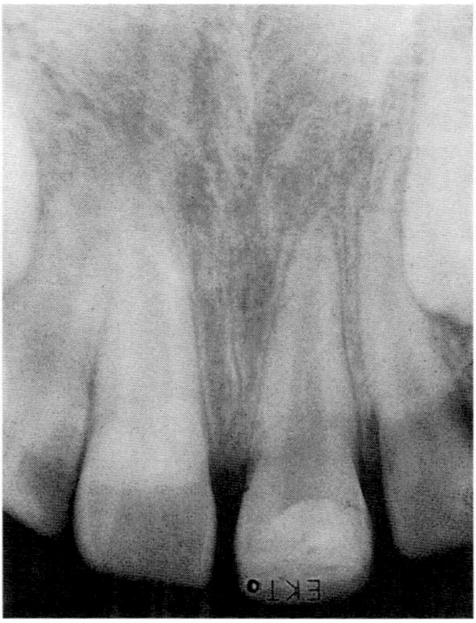

**Fig. 147** Enamel dentine fracture. Continued development and maturity of tooth in Fig. 146.

## Permanent tooth trauma I: reattachment of crown fragments

*Definition*

Reattachment to the tooth (immediately or delayed) of enamel dentine or minor enamel dentine pulp fractures.

*Clinical features and management*

Procedure is possible since the development of dentine bonding agents. If there is a minor pulp exposure then appropriate pulp treatment can be carried out, storing the fractured tooth fragment in normal saline – replenished weekly – until the pulp treatment is finished. The fragment is reattached using dentine bonding agent and composite resin as a luting cement (Figs 148, 149, 150).

*Complications*

- Few long-term follow-up studies.
- Opacity of the distal fragment.

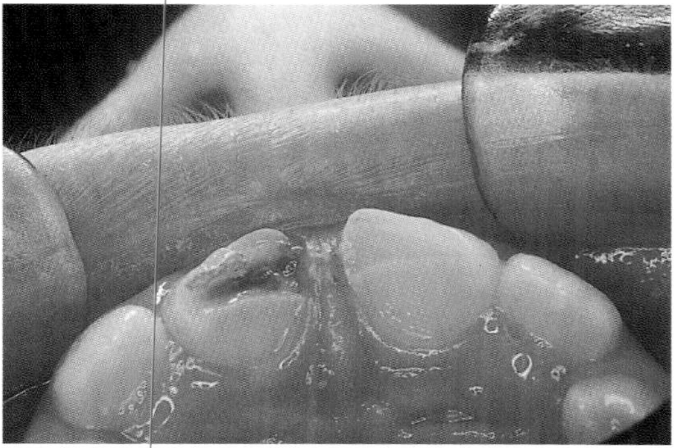

**Fig. 148** Enamel dentine and enamel dentine pulp fractures.

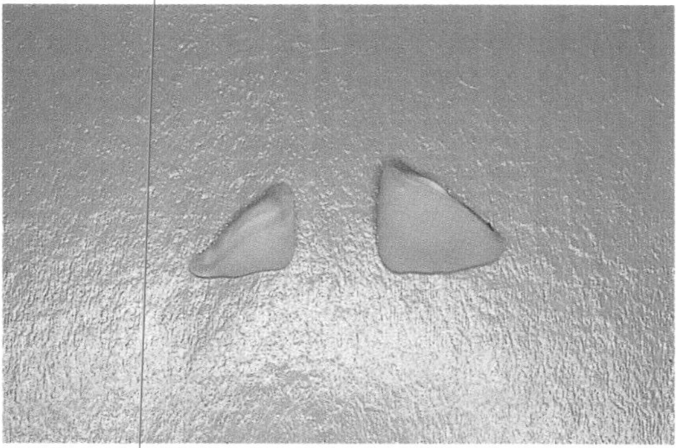

**Fig. 149** The tooth fragments from Fig. 148.

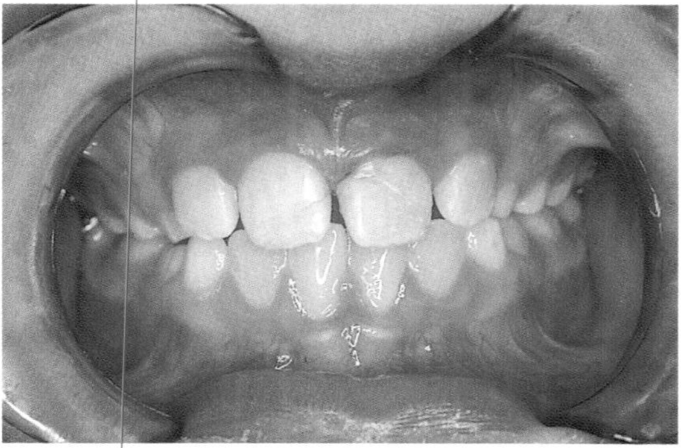

**Fig. 150** Fragments reattached.

## Permanent tooth trauma I: total or sub-total pulpotomy

*Definition*

Removal of all coronal pulp (pulpotomy) or 2–3 mm of the coronal pulp (sub-total pulpotomy) after a coronal fracture involving the pulp in a tooth with an immature (open) apex (Figs 151, 152).

*Investigations*

Periapical radiography to ascertain apical maturity initially and during follow-up.

Monitor the maturity of the width of the root canal as well as the apical maturity (Fig. 153).

*Clinical features*

The aim is to maintain radicular pulp vitality to enable complete root growth.

*Management*

- Remove coronal pulp with sharp excavators or slow running bur under LA and rubber dam.
- Place a layer of non-setting calcium hydroxide over the amputated pulp and cover with a restorative material that gives a hermetic seal.
- After 3 months, investigate for dentine bridge. If the bridge is present and there are no signs of periapical infection on radiography, then restore.
- If no bridge is present and there are signs of infection, proceed to induced apical closure.

*Complications*

Pulp necrosis of retained radicular pulp.

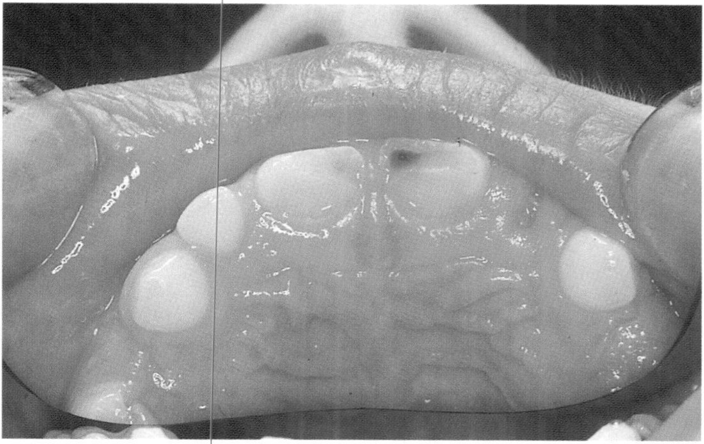

**Fig. 151** Enamel dentine pulp and enamel dentine fractures in teeth with immature roots.

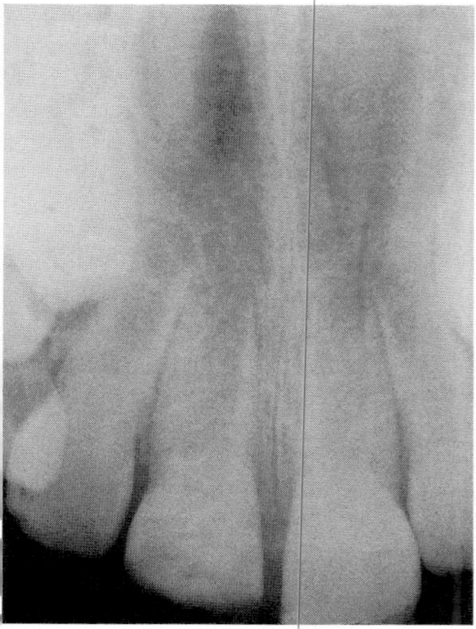

**Fig. 152** Pulpotomy: early treatment (different case to Fig. 151).

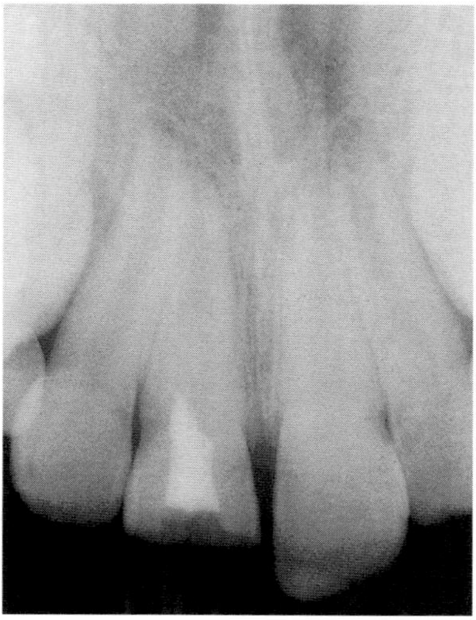

**Fig. 153** Pulpotomy: full root growth with vital radicular pulp (same case as Fig. 152).

## Permanent tooth trauma I: induced apical closure

*Definition*

Removal of non-vital pulp in a tooth with an immature (open) apex and placement into the root canal of non-setting calcium hydroxide cement to induce apical closure.

*Investigations*

Periapical radiography to ascertain apical maturity and to calculate the working length of the canal. Subsequent radiographs should assess the extent of apical closure.

*Clinical features*

To induce apical closure which will allow adequate obturation of the canal with gutta percha.

*Management*

Remove pulp under local anaesthetic and rubber dam. File canal. Working length is 1 mm short of radiographic apex (Fig. 154). Dry canal. Spin non-setting calcium hydroxide into the canal to the working length (Fig. 155). Review and change the non-setting calcium hydroxide 3–6 monthly. Average time to apical closure is 1 year. Obturate with gutta percha when apical closure has occurred (Figs 156, 157).

*Complications*

Non-closure. Obturation will be difficult by either the orthograde or the retrograde route.

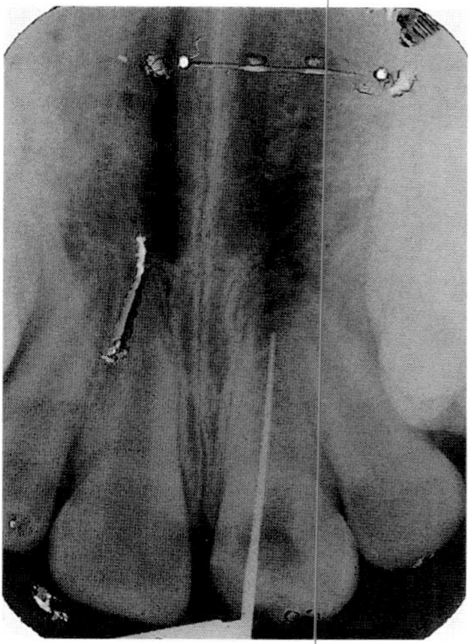

Fig. 154 Working length calculation.

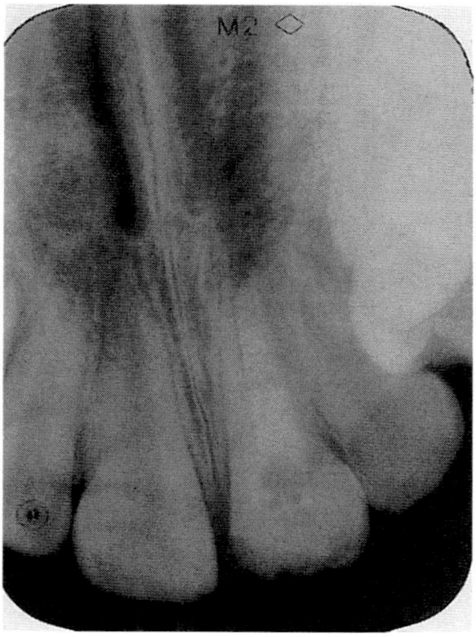
Fig. 155 Non-setting calcium hydroxide in root canal.

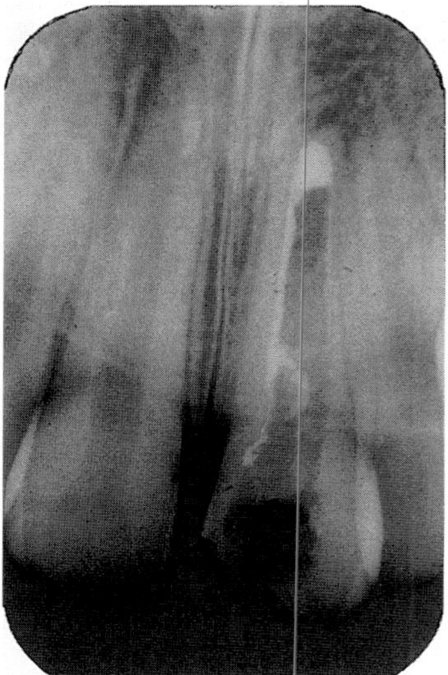
Fig. 156 Obturation of apical canal.

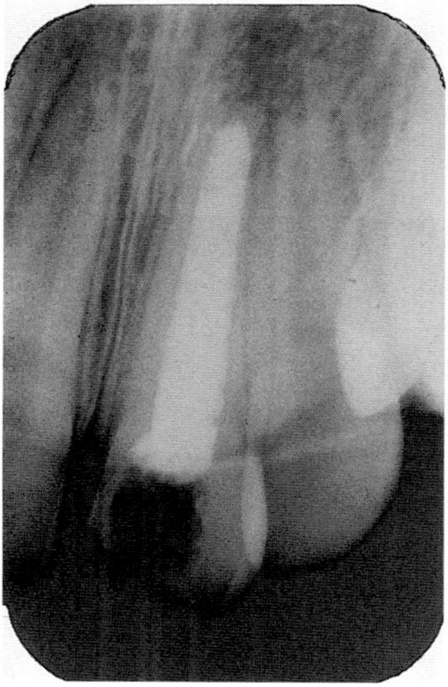
Fig. 157 Final obturation.

# 31 / Permanent tooth trauma II

## Root fractures

*Classification* Apical, middle, coronal thirds.

*Clinical features* Mobility; displacement of the coronal fragment; 'cracked cup' sound on percussion; tenderness to percussion.

*Investigations* Radiography. Anterior occlusal views often show root fractures more clearly than periapical views (Figs 158, 159).

*Management* Reduction of the displaced fragment and functional splinting for 2–3 weeks. Pulp treatment, if required, to the fracture line only. Leave the apical fragment alone as it often resorbs or undergoes intracanal calcification. Three types of healing are possible at the fracture line: calcified tissue; connective tissue; osteoid tissue.

*Complications* Coronal fractures have poor prognosis to heal. Removal of a mobile coronal fragment leaves three choices; immediate post and core after gingivoplasty; root extrusion and gingivoplasty followed by post and core; burial of the obturated root to maintain the height and width of the alveolar ridge for future implant.

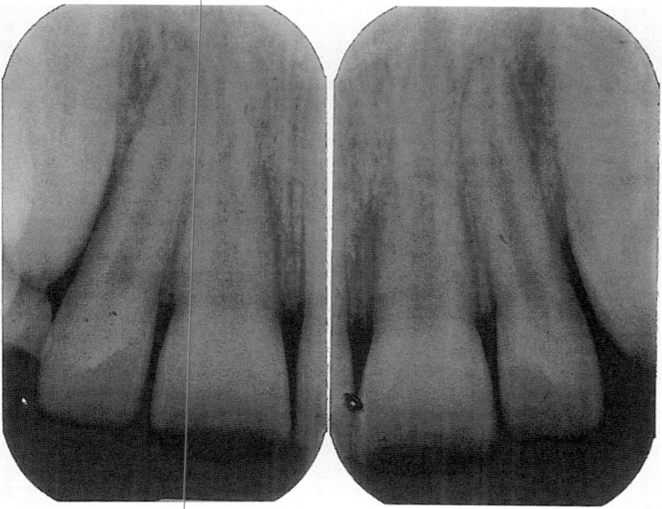

**Fig. 158** Root fractures: indistinct on periapical view.

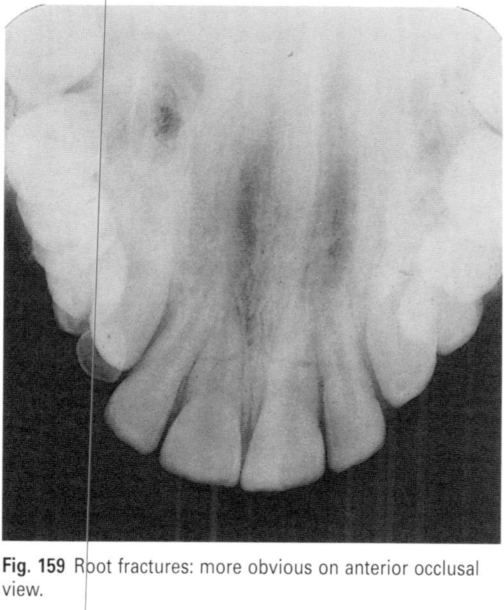

**Fig. 159** Root fractures: more obvious on anterior occlusal view.

## Permanent tooth trauma II: periodontal ligament injuries

*Definition*

*Concussion.* No abnormal loosening or displacement but marked reaction to percussion.

*Subluxation.* Abnormal loosening but no displacement.

*Extrusion.* Partial displacement of tooth from socket.

*Lateral luxation.* Displacement other than intrusion with comminution or fracture of alveolar socket (Fig. 160).

*Intrusion.* Displacement of tooth into the alveolus (Fig. 161).

*Avulsion.* Complete displacement of tooth from socket (Fig. 162).

*Management*

Specific management for each definition will differ, but all are covered by the following empirical categories:

- Reduction/replacement of the tooth to its normal position either manually or orthodontically.
- Splinting for a defined period (see p. 127).
- Regular clinical and radiographic review to determine the need for endodontics.

*Complications*

Pulp necrosis. Root resorption.

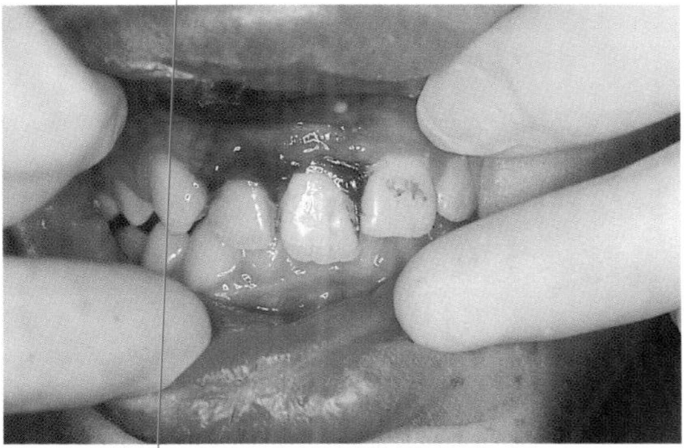

Fig. 160 Palatal luxation injury.

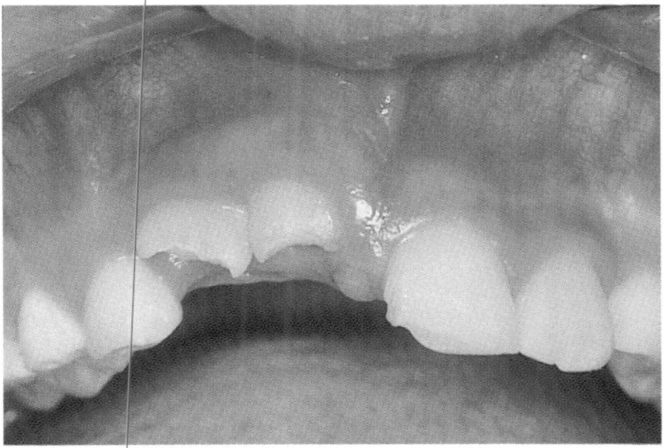

Fig. 161 Intrusion injury.

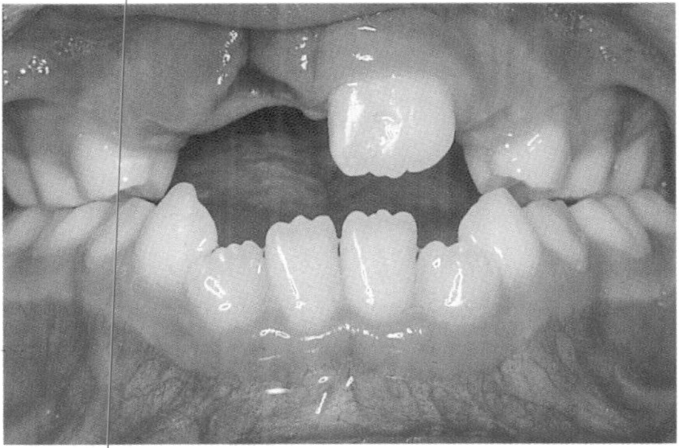

Fig. 162 Avulsion injury.

## Permanent tooth trauma II: dentoalveolar fractures

*Definition*

Fracture of the alveolar bone involving the tooth sockets.

*Clinical features*

A number of teeth are 'carried' on the fractured alveolus, producing an obvious step deformity in the dental arch (Fig. 163).

*Differential diagnosis*

Bilateral complete mandibular fractures through the lower border of the mandible.

*Investigations*

Periapical, lower occlusal and DPT radiography.

*Management*

- Reduction of the fracture (Fig. 164).
- Splinting for 3–4 weeks (Fig. 165).
- Antibiotic cover for 5 days (amoxycillin/erythromycin).
- Regular clinical and radiographic review of pulp vitality.

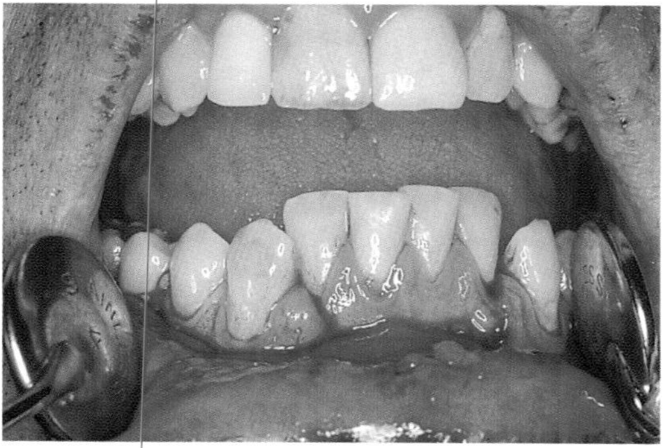

**Fig. 163** Displaced dentoalveolar fracture.

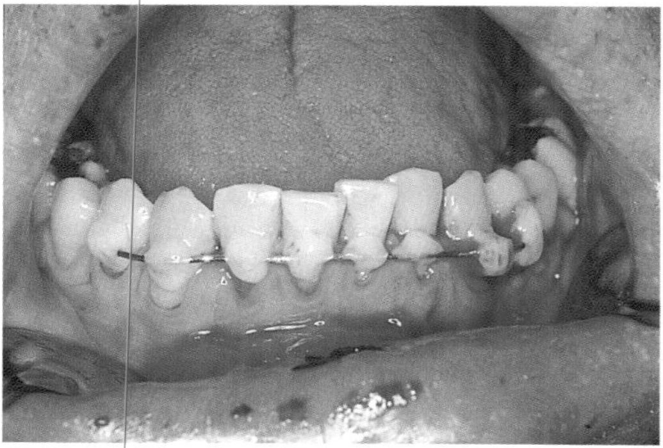

**Fig. 164** Reduced and splinted dentoalveolar fracture.

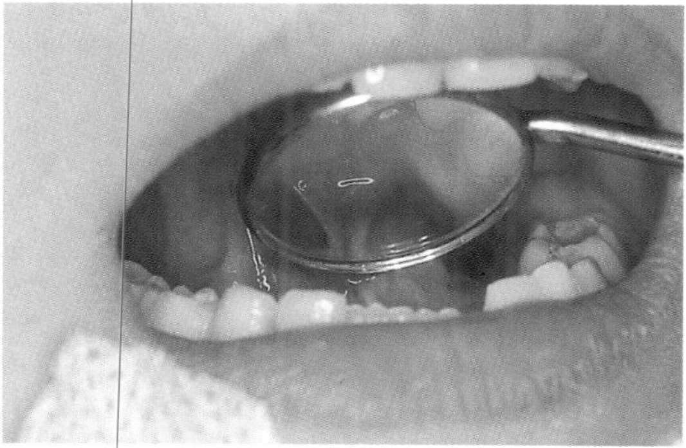

**Fig. 165** Sublingual haematoma in a dentoalveolar fracture.

## Splinting

Splinting is necessary in most periodontal ligament injuries to allow the fibres to heal. 60% of fibres are healed by 10–14 days. With the exception of dentoalveolar fractures which are splinted rigidly, all other injuries should have functional splints which allow some movement and prevent replacement resorption or ankylosis.

*Definition*

*Functional splint.* 7–10 days. This allows some functional movement. If using a composite-wire splint, there should be only one abutment tooth on either side of the injured tooth. It is used in avulsion injuries.

*Functional splint.* 2–3 weeks. One abutment tooth either side of the injured tooth. It is used in root fractures, subluxation, luxation, intrusion and extrusion injuries.

*Rigid splint.* 3–4 weeks. Two abutment teeth either side of the injured tooth. It is used in dentoalveolar fractures.

*Classification*

*Foil/milk bottle top.* Filled with temporary cement. Useful for single-handed operators out of normal working hours (Fig. 166).

*Composite-wire.* Stainless steel wire is bent to the correct shape and 'spot welded' to the centre of the labial surface of the teeth with acid etched composite (Fig. 167).

*Temporary crown material/wire.* As above but using temporary crown material. It is more difficult to apply than composite but easier to remove.

*Thermoplastic suck-down mouthguard type.* This needs laboratory equipment to make. The patient can remove it to brush teeth.

*Acrylic plate.* This covers the occlusal surface of the upper teeth. It is useful for injuries to newly erupted upper centrals where there are no abutment anterior primary teeth.

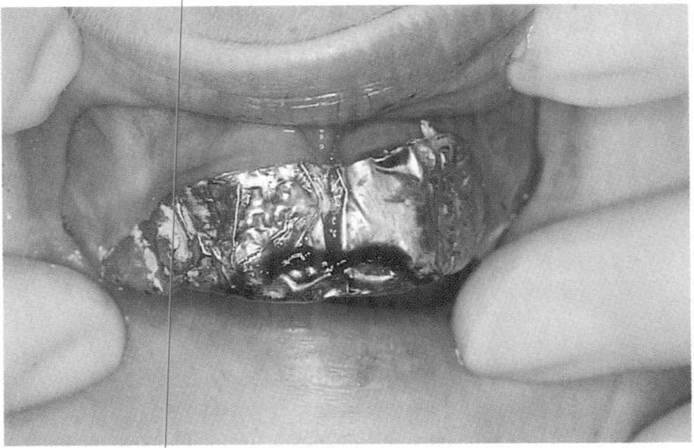

**Fig. 166** Temporary foil and cement splint.

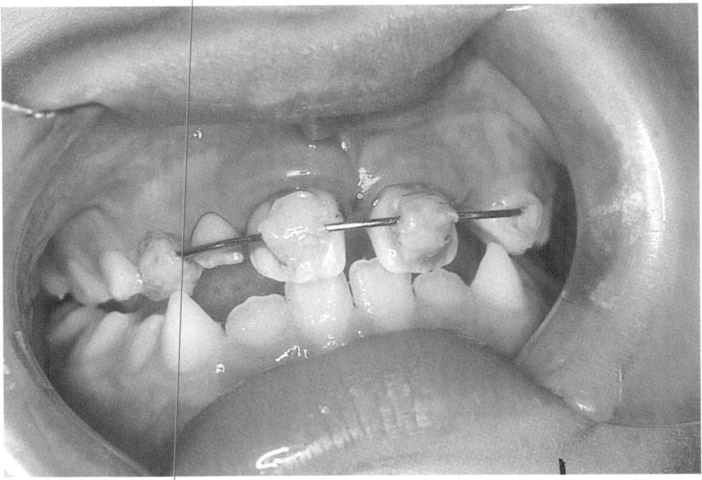

**Fig. 167** Composite-wire splint.

# Permanent tooth trauma III: soft tissue injuries

## Extraoral

*Management*

Facial swelling, bruises or lacerations may indicate underlying bony and tooth injury. Lacerations require careful debridement, to remove all foreign material, and suturing (Fig. 168). Antibiotics and/or tetanus toxoid may be required if wounds are contaminated.

Swollen lip with evidence of a penetrating wound, associated with a crown fracture, suggests retention of tooth fragments in the lip (Fig. 169). This may be clinically obvious (Fig. 169) or require radiographic localisation (Fig. 170).

## Intraoral

*Management*

Any lacerations should be examined for tooth fragments or foreign bodies.

Lacerations of lips or tongue require suturing but those of the oral mucosa heal very quickly and may not require suturing.

Antibiotics and/or tetanus toxoid may be required if wounds are contaminated.

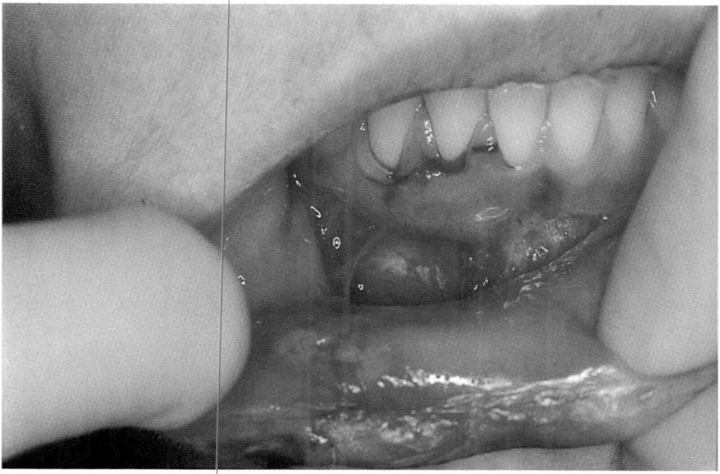

**Fig. 168** Degloving soft tissue injury.

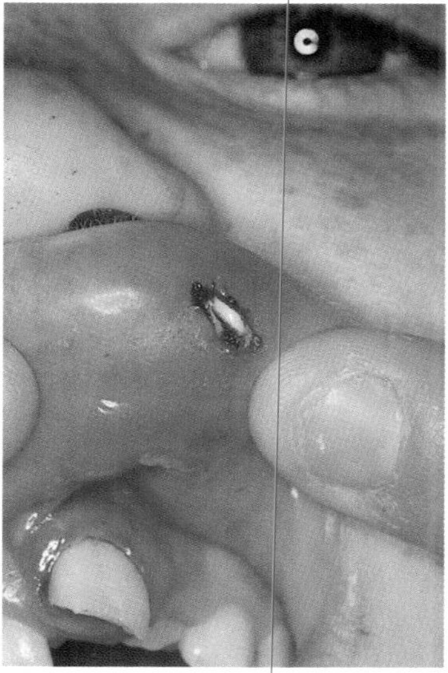

**Fig. 169** Tooth fragment in upper lip.

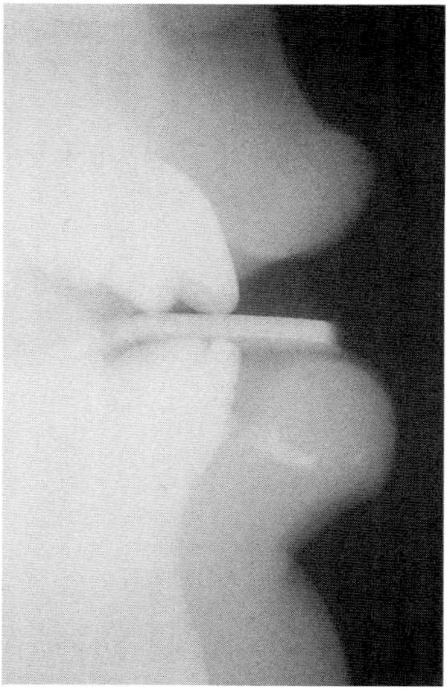

**Fig. 170** Tooth fragment in lower lip localised by radiography.

# Permanent tooth trauma III: resorption

## Internal resorption

| | |
|---|---|
| *Definition* | Resorption of the walls of the root canal giving the pulp space a ballooned appearance. External root surfaces are intact (Figs 171, 174). |
| *Aetiology* | Induction of multipotent pulpal cells into osteoclastic cells by necrotic pulp tissue. |
| *Differential diagnosis* | Other types of resorption. |
| *Investigations* | Clinical and radiographic assessment of pulpal and periodontal status. |
| *Management* | Pulpal extirpation followed by mechanical and chemical debridement of the root canal. Non-setting calcium hydroxide. Obturation with gutta percha when there is no progressive resorption. |

## External resorption

| | |
|---|---|
| *Definition* | Resorption of the external root surfaces to give an ill-defined 'punched-out' surface. Internal root canal surfaces are intact (Figs 172, 174). |
| *Aetiology* | Induction of multipotent periodontal ligament cells into osteoclastic cells by damage initially, and subsequently by pulpal necrotic products via dentinal tubules. |
| *Differential diagnosis* | Other types of resorption. |
| *Investigations* | Clinical and radiographic assessment of pulpal and periodontal status. |
| *Management* | Same as internal resorption. |

## Replacement resorption

| | |
|---|---|
| *Definition* | Loss of periodontal ligament and periodontal ligament space with direct union of cementum and bone (Figs 173, 174). |
| *Aetiology* | Extensive damage to PDL and cementum during luxation and avulsion injuries. |
| *Differential diagnosis* | Other types of resorption. |
| *Investigations* | Clinical and radiographic assessment of pulpal and periodontal status. |
| *Management* | Placement of non-setting calcium hydroxide into the root canal. If resorption is progressive, then plan for prosthetic replacement. |

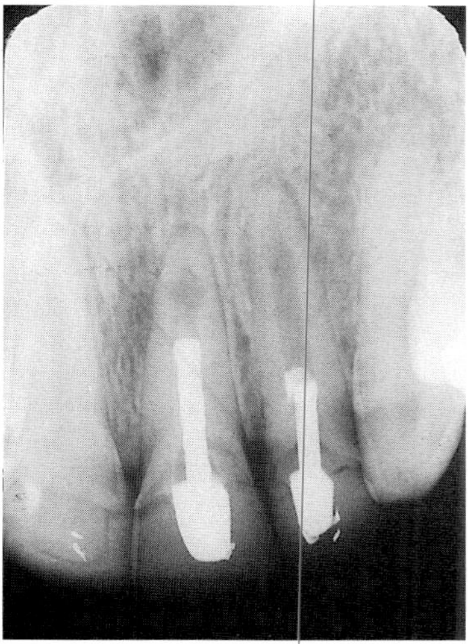

**Fig. 171** Internal resorption.

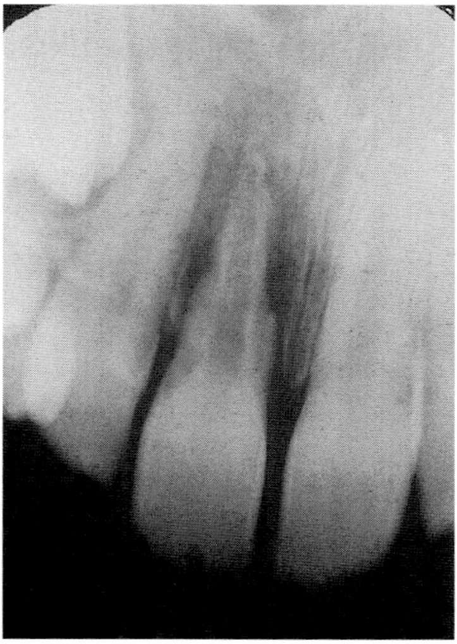

**Fig. 172** External inflammatory resorption.

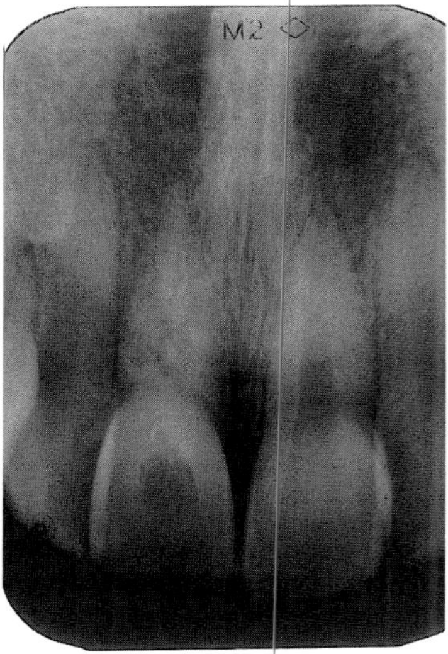


**Fig. 173** Replacement resorption.

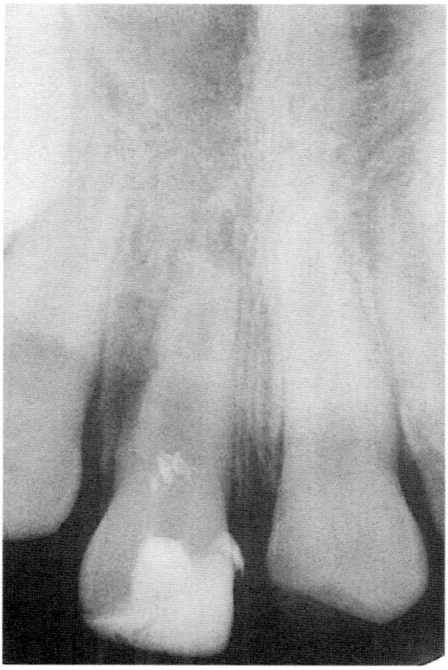

**Fig. 174** Mixture of internal, external and replacement resorption.

## Down syndrome

*Aetiology*

Trisomic chromosome anomaly usually involving chromosome 21. More prevalent in children born to elderly mothers. Incidence is 1 in 600 births.

*Clinical features*

Typical mongoloid appearance with brachycephaly and short stature; intellectual disability in nearly all cases; white spots (Brushfield's spots) around the iris (Fig. 175); single palmar crease (simian crease); clinodactyly of the fifth finger; macroglossia and fissured tongue; midface hypoplasia; microdontia; hypodontia; periodontal disease.

*Pathology*

50% have congenital cardiac defects. Multiple immune defects predispose to acute leukaemia, blepharitis, keratitis, upper respiratory infections, and periodontal disease.

*Management*

Antibiotic prophylaxis will be required if there is congenital cardiac disease. Aggressive prevention.

## Childhood cancer

*Incidence*

1 in 600 children under the age of 15 in the UK.

*Classification*

*Leukaemias.* Abnormal proliferation of white blood cells (48% of all childhood cancers).

*Solid tumours.* Affecting tissues: central nervous system 16%; lymphoma 8%; neuroblastoma 7%; nephroblastoma 5%; others 16% of all childhood cancers.

*Management*

Chemotherapy; radiotherapy; bone marrow transplant (Fig. 176).

*Complications*

*Immunosuppression.* Susceptibility to bacterial, viral and fungal infections.

*Haemorrhage.* No invasive dental procedures should be carried out until platelets are $80 \times 10^9$ g/l.

*Mortality rate.* 30–40%.

*Oral and dental complications.* Microdontia; hypodontia; thin roots; short roots; large pulp chambers; enamel hypoplasia; dry mouth (secondary to radiotherapy) (Fig. 177).

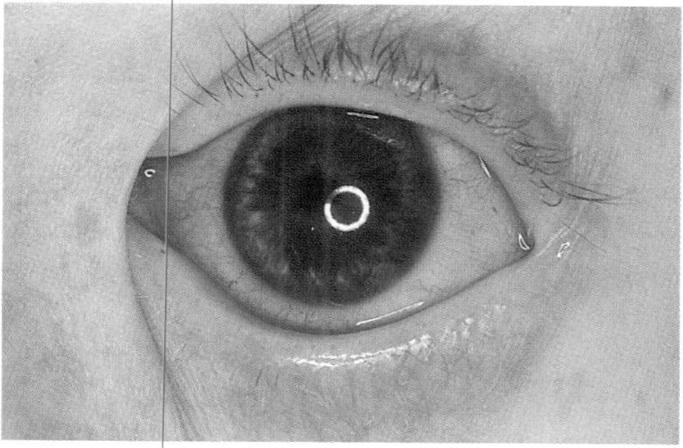

**Fig. 175** Brushfield's spots.

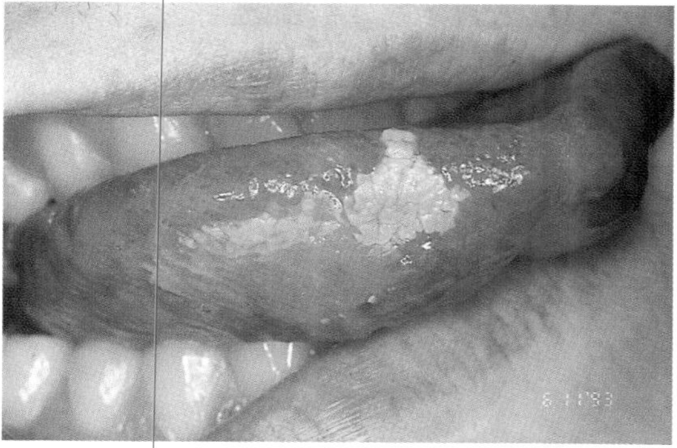

**Fig. 176** Leukoplakia in graft versus host disease after bone marrow transplantation.

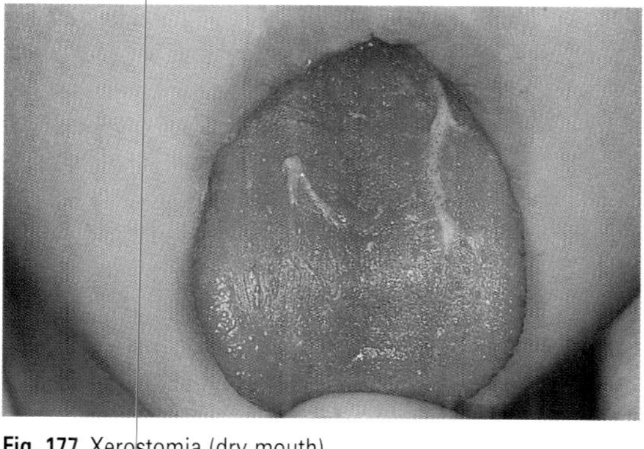

**Fig. 177** Xerostomia (dry mouth).

## Congenital cardiac disease

*Aetiology*

Multifactorial inheritance. Chromosomal abnormalities represent fewer than 5% of the total.

*Classification and prevalence*

Ventricular septal defect 28%; atrial septal defect 10%; pulmonary stenosis 10%; patent ductus arteriosus 10%; tetralogy of Fallot 10%; aortic stenosis 7%; coarctation of the aorta 5%; transposition of the great arteries 5%; rare/diverse 15%.

*Clinical features*

Shortness of breath, finger clubbing (Fig. 178), cyanosis (Fig. 179), recurrent respiratory infections, delayed growth and development.

*Management*

Antibiotic prophylaxis to prevent infective endocarditis. Some surgical cardiac procedures are completely curative. **Always check with cardiologist for the need for antibiotic cover**. Aggressive prevention.

*Complications*

Infective endocarditis has a 20% mortality.

## Bleeding disorders

*Definition*

Any disorder that upsets the normal: local reactions of the blood vessels; platelet activities; interaction of specific coagulation factors that circulate in the blood (Fig. 180).

*Classifications*

*Coagulation defects*
- Inherited: factor deficiency, e.g. VIII haemophilia A.
- Acquired: liver disease; vitamin deficiency; anticoagulant drugs.

*Thrombocytopenic purpura*
- Primary: lack of platelets, e.g. idiopathic thrombocytopenic purpura (ITP).
- Secondary: systemic disease, e.g. leukaemia; drug induced; radiation.

*Non-thrombocytopenic purpura*
- Vascular wall alteration: scurvy; infections; allergy.
- Disorders of platelet function: inherited von Willebrand's disease; drugs; allergy; autoimmune.

*Management*

Close liaison with medical colleagues essential. Aggressive prevention.

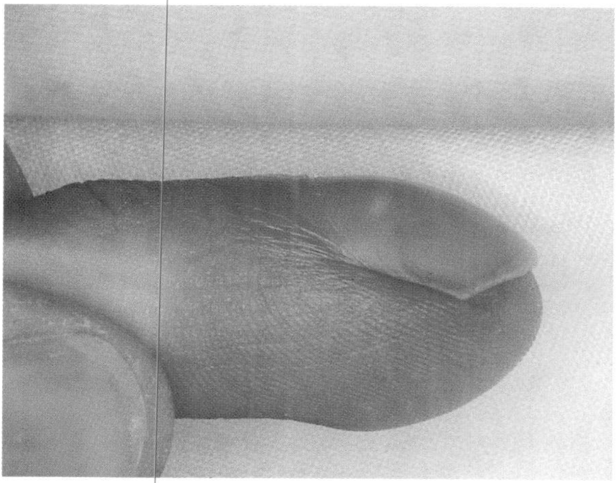

**Fig. 178** Finger clubbing.

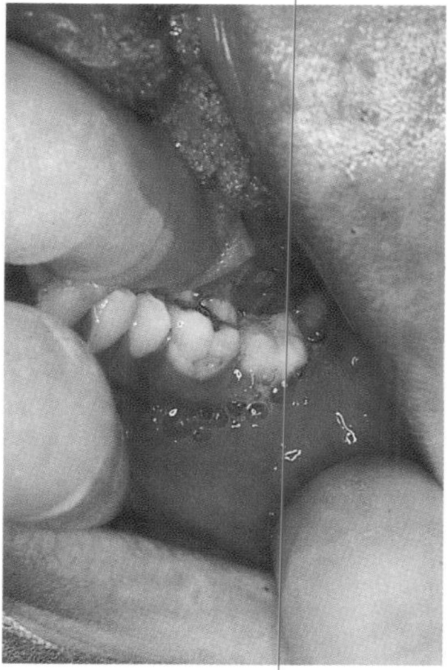

**Fig. 179** Cyanosis of oral mucosa.

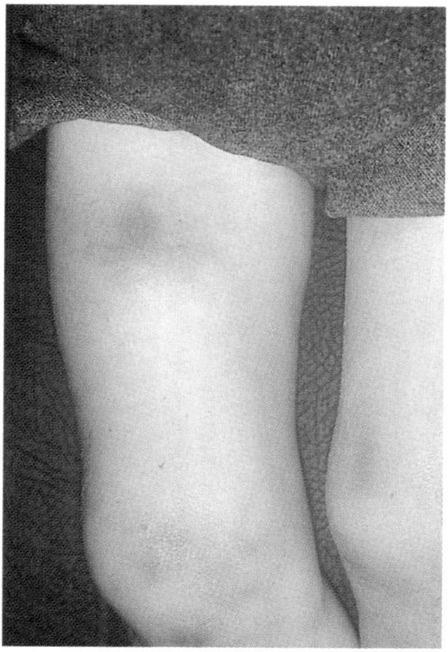

**Fig. 180** Deep haematoma in haemophilia A factor VIII deficiency.

## Primary herpetic gingivostomatitis

*Aetiology and pathology*

Occurs typically at age 2–4 years after an incubation period of 6–7 days. Usually caused by herpes simplex virus 1 (HSV-1).

*Diagnosis*

Gingival oedema, erythema and widespread oral vesiculation (Fig. 181). Areas of vesiculation break down and fuse to produce irregular, painful ulcers. Systemic features of malaise, fever and cervical lymphadenopathy. Saliva is heavily infected with HSV, which may cause lip and skin lesions and is a source of cross-infection.

*Management*

Rehydration, analgesia and systemic acyclovir.

## Secondary (recurrent) herpes labialis

*Aetiology and pathology*

HSV-1 lies dormant in the trigeminal ganglion. Labialis is caused by reactivation by fever, sunlight, trauma or immunosuppression. 6–14% of the population have recurrent herpes labialis.

*Diagnosis*

Macules develop at the mucocutaneous junction of the lip which progresses to papules and vesicles which become pustular, scab, and heal without scarring (Fig. 182).

*Management*

Topical acyclovir as soon as tingling is felt.

## Ocular herpes

*Aetiology and pathology*

HSV-1. Spread from primary or secondary lesion by finger.

*Diagnosis*

Corneal injection. Presence of oral lesions (Fig. 183).

*Management*

Self-limiting. Eye occlusion may be required if movement of the eyelids over the cornea is painful.

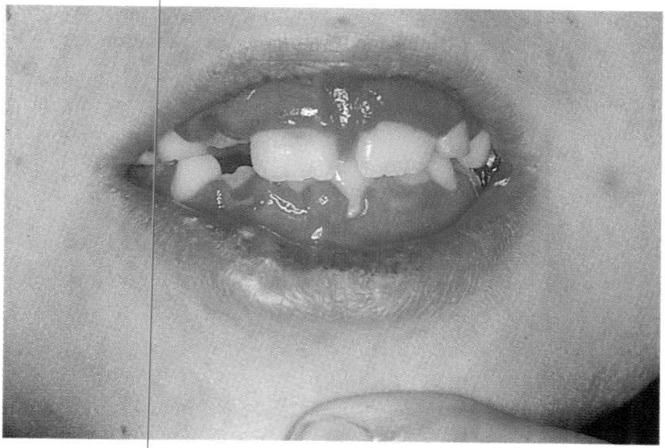

Fig. 181 Primary herpetic gingivostomatitis.

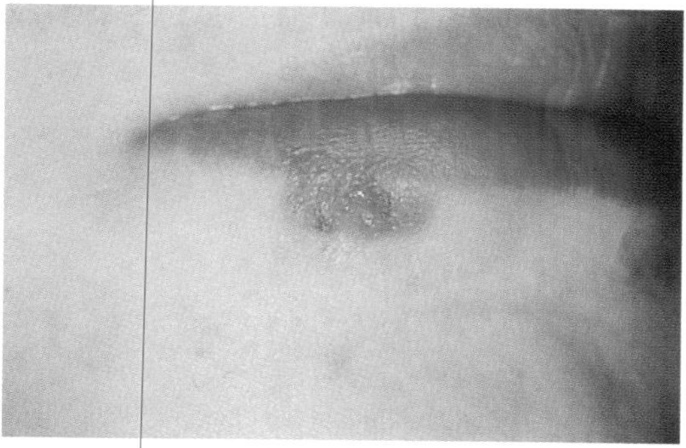

Fig. 182 Recurrent herpes labialis.

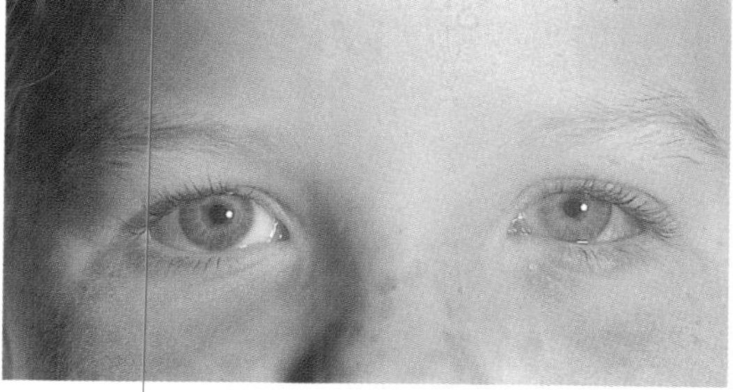

Fig. 183 Ocular herpes of the left eye.

## Herpes zoster

*Aetiology and pathology*

Herpes varicella zoster (HVZ) virus. More common in adults than in children.

*Diagnosis*

Vesicular lesion develops within the peripheral distribution of the trigeminal or cervical nerves (Fig. 184).

*Management*

Analgesia.

## Hand-foot-and-mouth disease

*Aetiology and pathology*

Coxsackie A virus infection (commonly A-16).

*Diagnosis*

- Small, painful vesicles surrounded by inflammatory haloes, especially on the dorsum and lateral aspect of the fingers and toes.
- Rash is not always present.
- May also affect more proximal limbs (Fig. 185) or buttocks.
- Oral lesions are shallow, painful, small and surrounded by inflammatory haloes.

*Management*

Supportive.

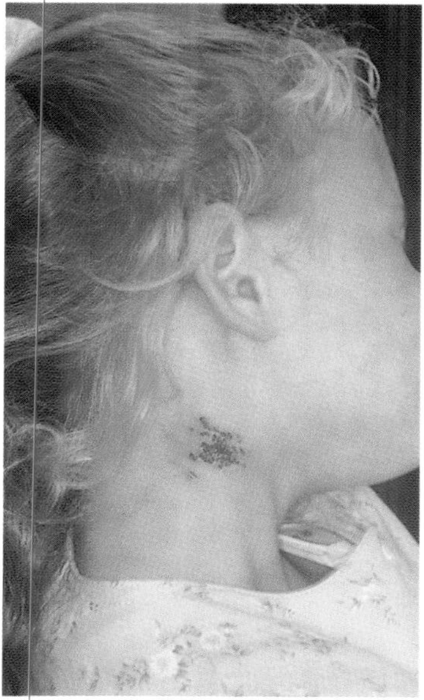

**Fig. 184** Herpes zoster of the cervical region.

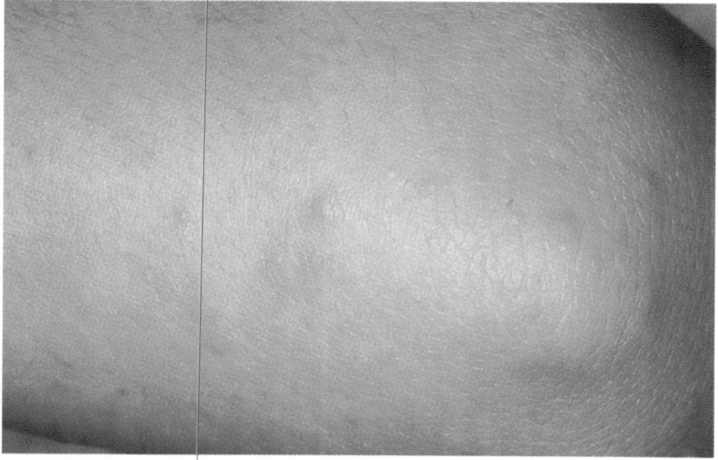

**Fig. 185** Hand-foot-and-mouth disease around the elbow.

# 35 / Aphthae

The main causes of mouth ulcers in children are:

- Local causes (e.g. trauma)
- Recurrent aphthae
- Associated with systemic disease (e.g. coeliac disease)
- Drugs (e.g. cytotoxics)
- Irradiation of the mucosa.

## Recurrent aphthous stomatitis (RAS)

*Aetiology and pathology*

20% of children may have a haematinic deficiency. 1–3% may have coeliac disease. A smaller number may be hypersensitive to food constituents. 40% of those with RAS have a family history. It may be precipitated by trauma, stress, or illness.

*Diagnosis*

Small (2–4 mm) in diameter, last 7–10 days, tend not to occur on gingiva, palate and dorsum of the tongue (Figs 186, 187), and heal without scarring.

*Management*

- Eliminate haematinic deficiency, systemic illness or hypersensitivity.
- Symptomatic application of antibacterial/steroid preparations.

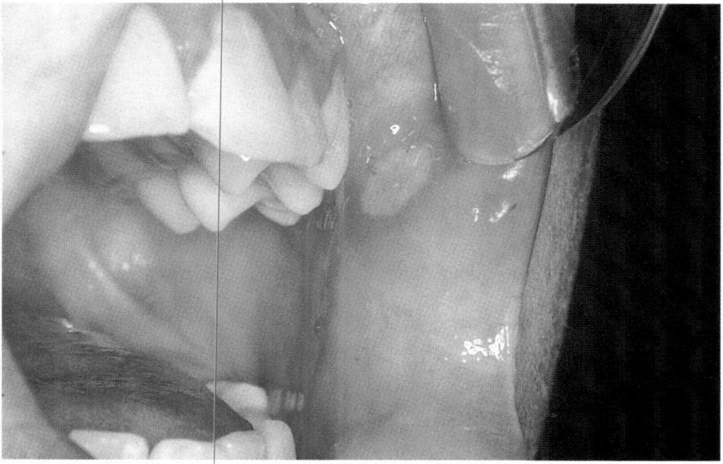

**Fig. 186** Recurrent aphthous stomatitis.

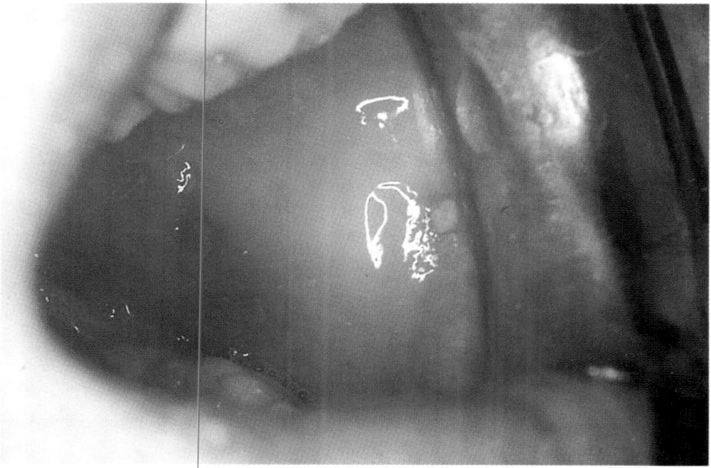

**Fig. 187** Recurrent aphthous stomatitis.

## Acute necrotising ulcerative gingivitis (ANUG)

*Aetiology and pathology*

Fusospirochaetal complex together with Gram-negative anaerobic organisms including *Porphyromonas gingivalis*, *Veillonella* and *Selenomonas* species.

In developing countries it may affect children as young as 1–2 years.

In developed countries it commonly affects people in the 16–30 age range.

*Diagnosis*

Necrosis and ulceration affecting interdental papilla which then spreads to labial and lingual marginal gingiva. 'Punched out' appearance (Fig. 188).

*Management*

Oral hygiene, mouth rinses with chlorhexidine 0.2%, hydrogen peroxide or sodium hydroxyperborate mouth rinse, antibiotics effective against anaerobes (e.g. metronidazole).

## Chronic gingivitis

*Aetiology and pathology*

Inflammatory infiltrate in response to the accumulation of dental plaque next to the gingival margin. Early flora in plaque are Gram-positive cocci after 4–7 days, followed by filamentous and fusiform Gram-negative organisms after 2 weeks.

*Diagnosis*

Swelling and erythema of gingival margins. Bleeding on brushing or eating. Halitosis (Figs. 189, 190).

*Management*

Toothbrush instruction. Initial use of chlorhexidine 0.2% mouthwash.

If left untreated it will progress to periodontitis.

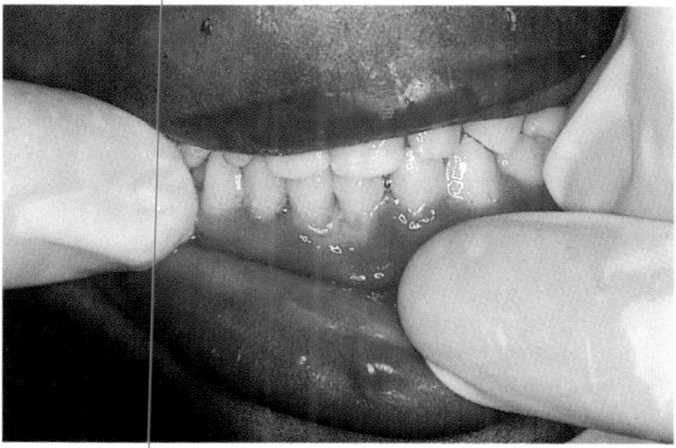

**Fig. 188** Acute necrotising ulcerative gingivitis in the primary dentition.

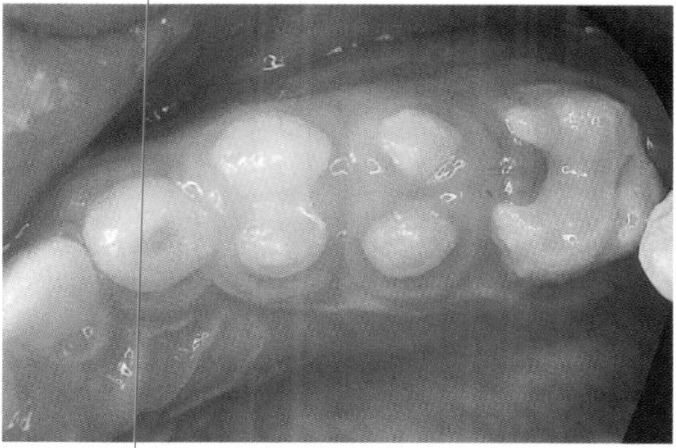

**Fig. 189** Chronic gingivitis around newly erupting teeth.

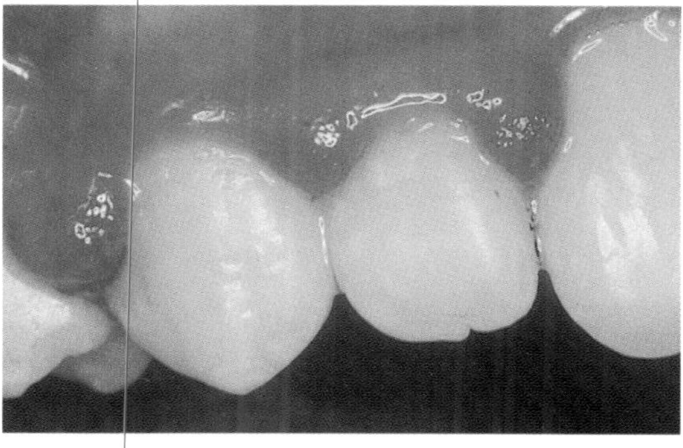

**Fig. 190** Chronic gingivitis of upper labial gingiva.

# 37 / Periodontitis

Chronic periodontitis is rare in young children but can be associated with poor nutrition, previous acute necrotising ulcerative gingivitis and HIV. In older children periodontitis will progress from marginal gingivitis if plaque removal is not efficient. Localised juvenile periodontitis (prepubertal periodontitis) is rare but occurs in the presence of good plaque control and may be related to an immune defect. Systemic conditions may underlie periodontitis: diabetes mellitus (Fig. 191); white cell defects and neutropenias; Down syndrome.

## Localised juvenile periodontitis

*Aetiology and pathology* — Microorganisms: *Actinobacillus (Haemophilus) actinomycetemcomitans* and *Capnocytophaga.*

*Diagnosis* — Localised periodontal destruction, classically in the permanent incisor and first molar regions (Fig. 191).

*Management* — Tooth brushing instruction, root planing, local and systemic antibiotics.

## Neutrophil defects and neutropenias

*Aetiology and pathology* — Either abnormal function or reduced numbers of neutrophils.

*Diagnosis* — Progressive periodontal destruction in the presence of good oral hygiene (Figs 192, 193). Early tooth loss.

*Management* — Good oral hygiene and use of chlorhexidine 0.2% will help to maintain teeth for as long as possible.

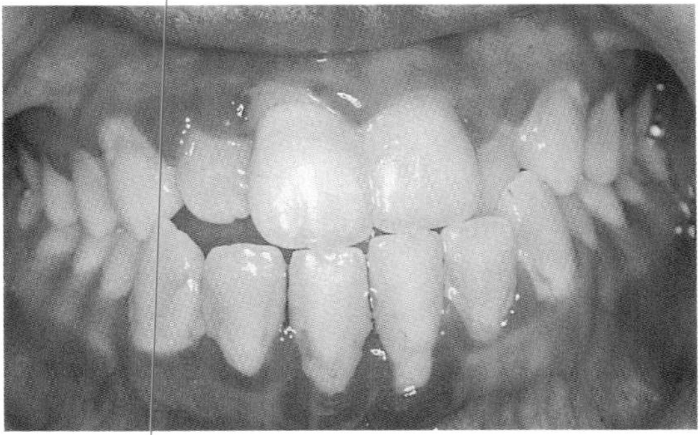

**Fig. 191** Juvenile periodontitis in a teenager with diabetes mellitus.

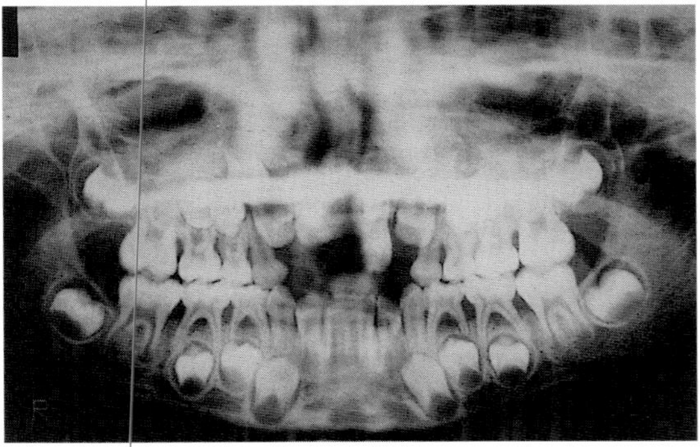

**Fig. 192** Chronic periodontitis in a 6-year-old child with cyclical neutropenia.

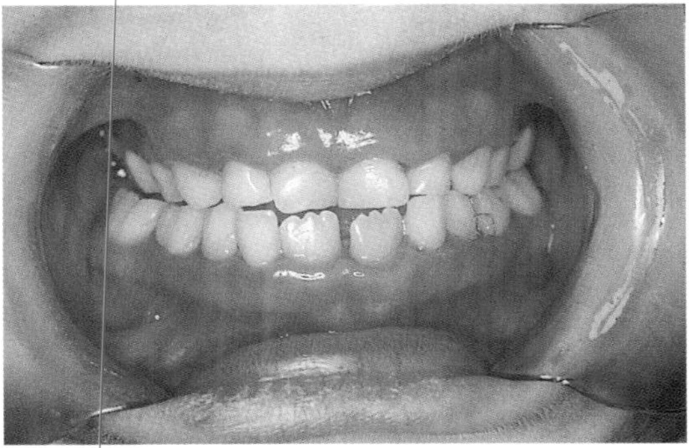

**Fig. 193** Clinical appearance of the patient in Fig. 192.

## Gingivitis artefacta

*Aetiology and pathology*
Self-induced, usually with fingernail.

*Diagnosis*
Labial surface of tooth commonly (Fig. 194). Identification of habit.

*Management*
Reassurance. Progressive damage in those with an intellectual disability may require protection in the form of a splint.

## Localised recession

*Aetiology and pathology*
Narrow zone of keratined gingiva (e.g. when teeth erupt labially to their predecessors). Aggravating factors such as gingivitis or mechanical irritation from excessive and incorrect toothbrushing may exacerbate recession.

*Diagnosis*
Characteristic appearance (Fig. 195).

*Management*
*Conservative.* Record the maximum distance from the gingival margin to cementum – enamel junction. Correct abnormal toothbrushing. Monitor into adolescence as attachment will creep coronally spontaneously.

*Surgical.* Guided tissue regeneration or other muco-gingival surgery.

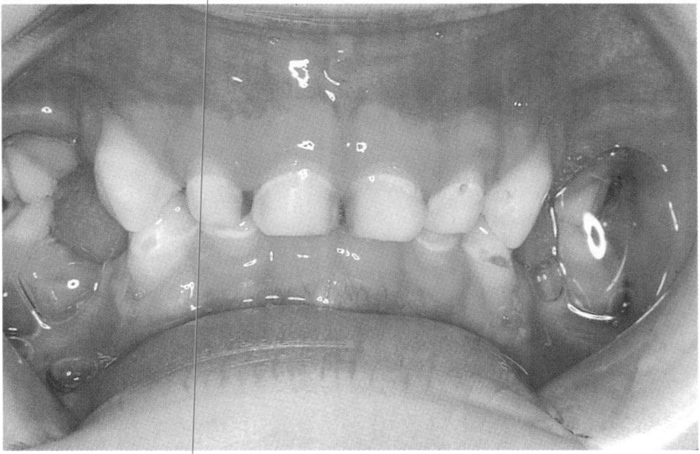

**Fig. 194** Gingivitis artefacta: gingival recession in the upper and lower canine regions.

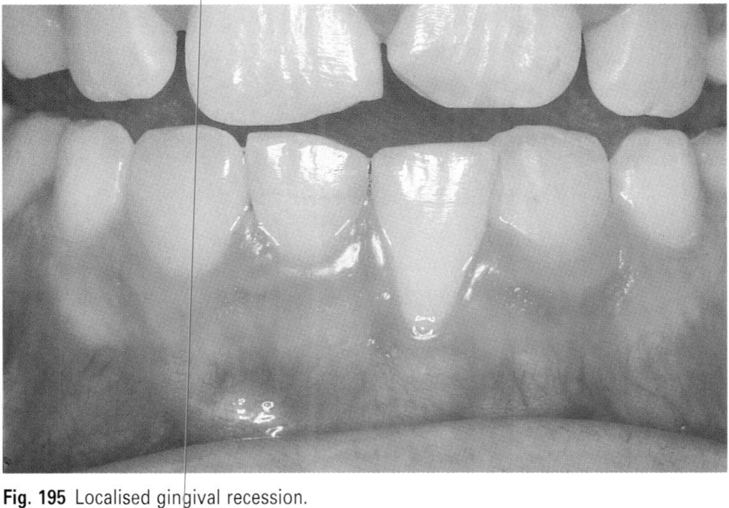

**Fig. 195** Localised gingival recession.

# 39 / Gingival overgrowth

## Localised gingival hyperplasia

*Aetiology and pathology* — Hyperplastic response to inadequate local oral hygiene.

*Diagnosis* — Localised hyperplasia in the presence of chronic gingivitis and plaque accumulation (Fig. 196).

*Management* — Toothbrush instruction followed by localised surgery.

## Drug-induced gingival overgrowth

*Aetiology and pathology* — Side-effect of a number of drugs. The commonest are: phenytoin (anticonvulsant); cyclosporin (immunosuppressant); nifedipine (antihypertensive).

Exacerbated by poor oral hygiene.

*Diagnosis* — Firm, progressive gingival hyperplasia with a drug history (Fig. 197).

*Management* — Surgery when oral hygiene is satisfactory. Overgrowth will recur if the drug treatment continues.

## Hereditary gingival fibromatosis

*Aetiology and pathology* — Familial condition associated with hirsutism (Fig. 198). Rare associations occur with epilepsy, sensorineural deafness and some syndromes. Histological analysis shows dense collagenous hyperplasia.

*Diagnosis* — Family history. Often apparent when permanent teeth erupt. Generalised firm gingival enlargement.

*Management* — Gingival surgery. Slow regrowth will occur.

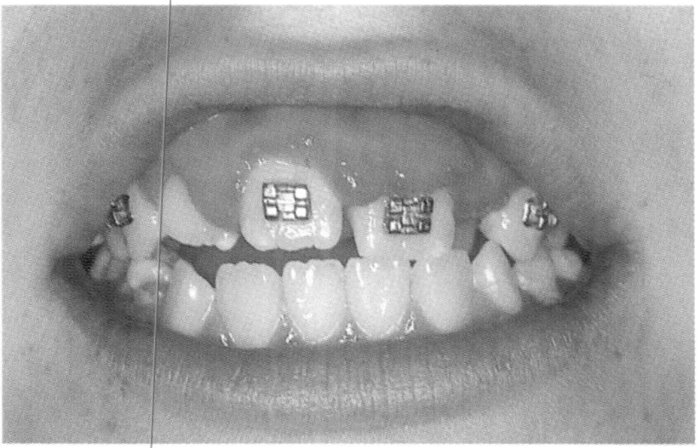

**Fig. 196** Localised gingival overgrowth associated with upper incisors.

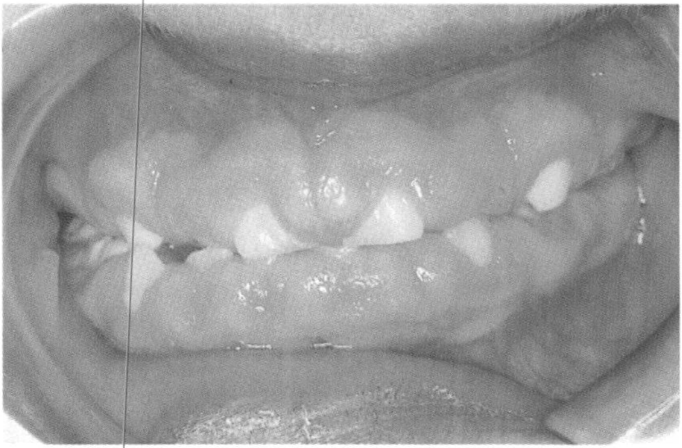

**Fig. 197** Drug-induced gingival overgrowth.

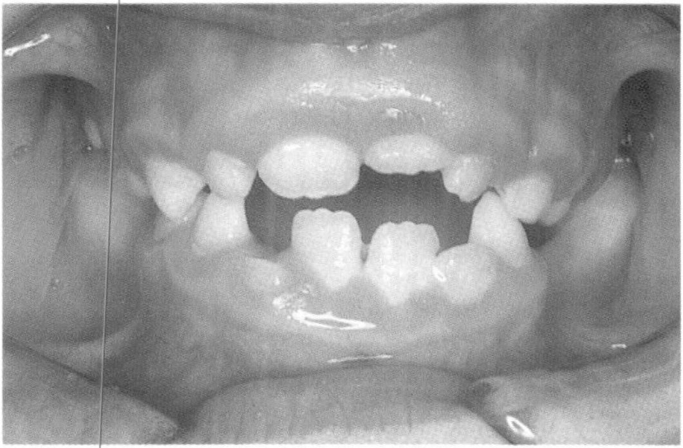

**Fig. 198** Hereditary gingival fibromatosis.

## Granulomas

### Pyogenic granuloma

*Aetiology and pathology*

Commonly affects the gingiva, lip or tongue and is an exaggerated response to minor trauma. Pyogenic granulomas are soft, fleshy, rough-surfaced, vascular lesions that bleed readily and are usually seen on the buccal aspect of the interdental papilla of the anterior gingiva (Fig. 199).

Plaque accumulation, calculus, or carious cavitation are common irritants.

*Diagnosis*

Characteristic swelling in the presence of irritants and histological examination.

*Management*

- Improved oral hygiene and restoration of carious lesions.
- Surgical removal of lesion (Fig. 200).

### Giant cell granuloma (giant cell epulis)

*Aetiology and pathology*

Non-neoplastic swelling of proliferating fibroblasts in a highly vascular stroma containing multinucleate giant cells. Characteristically occur adjacent to permanent teeth that have predecessors (Fig. 201). They are often a deep red colour. Older lesions may be paler.

*Diagnosis*

Characteristic swelling and histological examination.

*Management*

Surgical excision. The condition requires clinical follow-up as recurrence is common. It may be a feature of hyperparathyroidism.

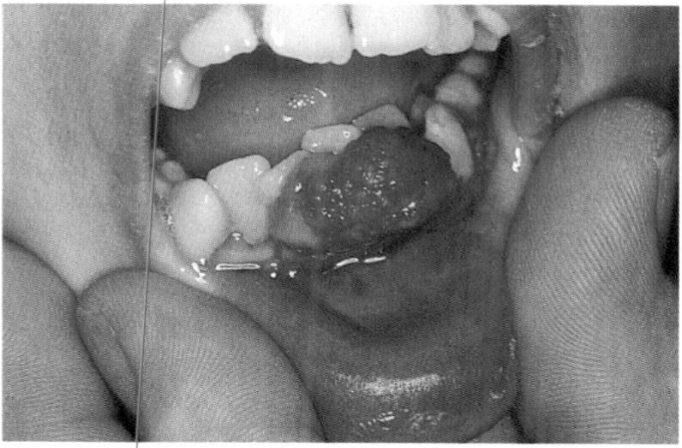

**Fig. 199** Pyogenic granuloma.

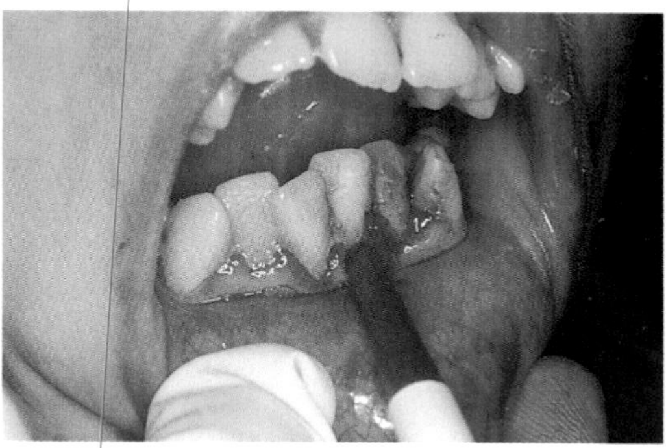

**Fig. 200** Calculus and staining are visible after pyogenic granuloma removal.

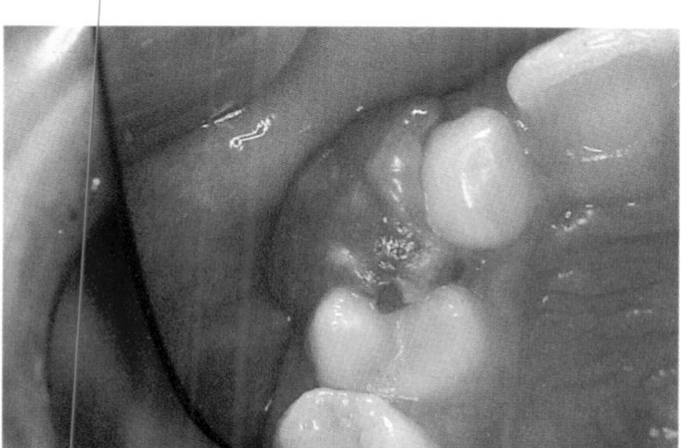

**Fig. 201** Giant cell granuloma on the labial aspect of the upper alveolus.

# Traumatic lesions I

### Fibroepithelial polyp

*Aetiology and pathology*
Chronic trauma, usually from biting, resulting in fibrous hyperplasia (Fig. 202).

*Diagnosis*
Differentiate from other soft tissue lesions by histological examination of the excised lesion.

*Management*
Excisional biopsy and histological confirmation.

### Mucocele

*Aetiology and pathology*
Most are caused by saliva extravasation into the tissues from damage to minor salivary gland ducts. They are commonly seen in the lower labial and ventral lingual mucosa (Fig. 203).

*Diagnosis*
History of trauma and characteristic appearance.

*Management*
Surgical removal may be required if there is regular trauma. Recurrence may occur.

### Ranula

*Aetiology and pathology*
A mucocele that occurs from the sublingual gland. Blue transparent appearance (Fig. 204).

*Diagnosis*
Characteristic appearance and location.

*Management*
Excision of the sublingual gland.

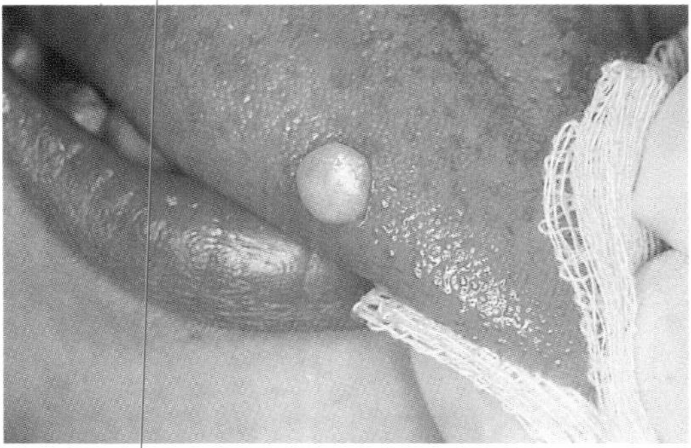

Fig. 202 Fibroepithelial polyp.

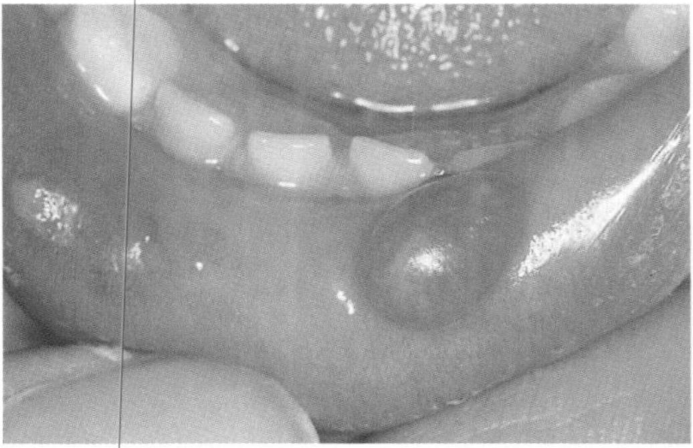

Fig. 203 Mucocele.

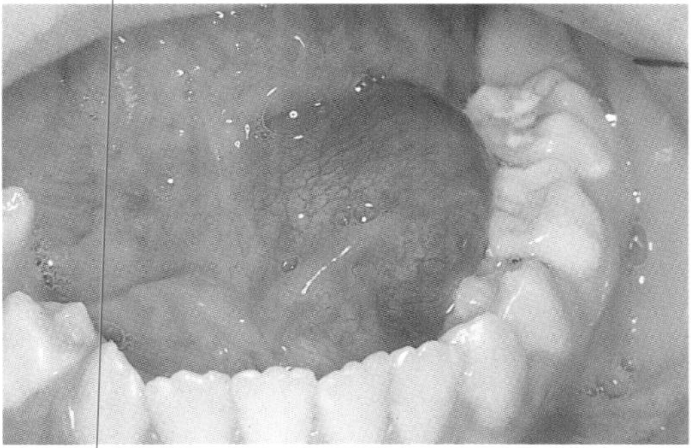

Fig. 204 Ranula.

# Traumatic lesions II

## Burns

*Aetiology and pathology*

Most common after the ingestion of hot foods and are seen particularly on the palate or tongue. Other causes are cotton-wool when it is removed from the sulcus quickly, analgesic tablets positioned on the mucosa next to a painful tooth, and chemicals used in restorative dentistry (Fig. 205).

*Diagnosis*

Characteristic sites related to eating, restoration of a tooth, or a painful tooth.

*Management*

Reassurance that healing will occur without scarring.

Topical local anaesthetic may help.

## Sharp teeth and restorations

*Aetiology and pathology*

The normal mammelons on newly erupted lower incisors may produce frictional trauma to the tongue (Fig. 206). This is often worse if the child has a physical or intellectual disability. Sharp restorations have a similar effect.

*Diagnosis*

Lesion is site specific and related to a sharp edge.

*Management*

Smooth the edge, apply an adhesive restorative material, or make a soft 'blow down' splint.

## Local anaesthetic

*Aetiology and pathology*

Biting the area of anaesthetised mucosa.

*Diagnosis*

Confined to the area of anaesthetised mucosa (Fig. 207).

*Management*

Reassurance. May require antibiotics if the bitten area becomes secondarily infected.

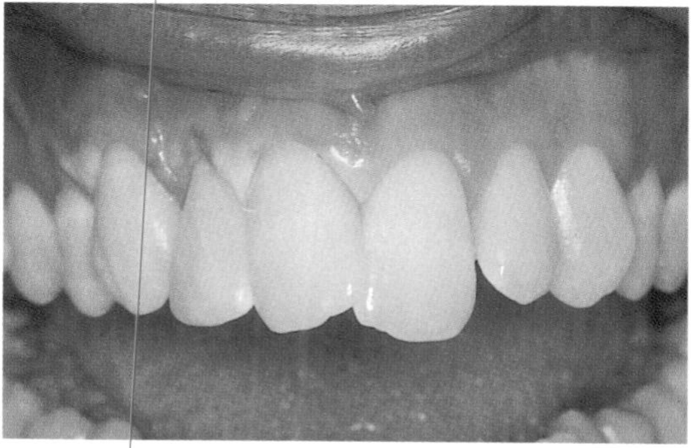

Fig. 205 Dentine primer burn of the upper gingiva.

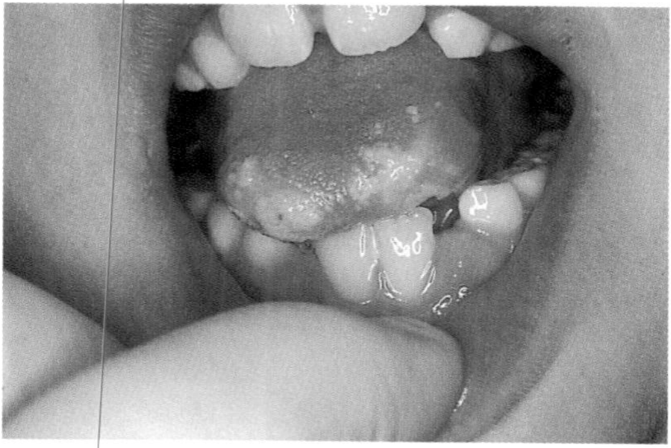

Fig. 206 Frictional trauma of the tongue from the mammelons on the lower central incisors.

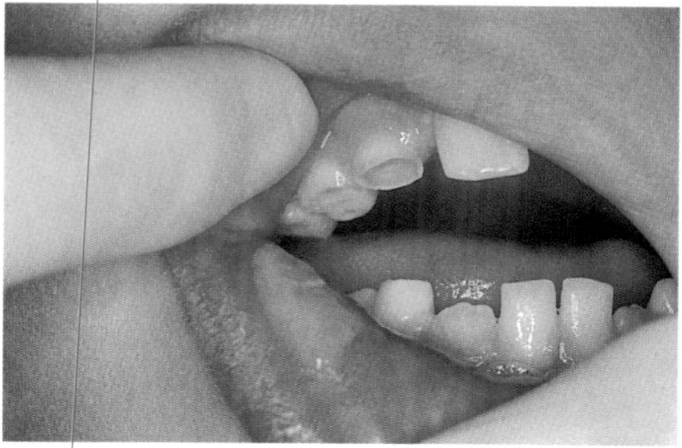

Fig. 207 Ulcer from biting anaesthetised mucosa.

# 41 / Assorted mucosal lesions

## Geographic tongue

*Aetiology and pathology*

A benign condition of unknown aetiology affecting up to 1.5% of the population. Irregular desquamation of filiform papillae in a demarcated pattern (Fig. 208). It often exists together with scrotal or fissured tongue, which is more frequent in Down syndrome or Melkersson–Rosenthal syndrome.

*Diagnosis*

Demarcated pattern which changes with time.

*Management*

Reassurance. Avoid spicy and salty foods.

## Lichen planus

*Aetiology and pathology*

Rare in children but may be associated with non-steroidal anti-inflammatory agents, antimalarial drugs, some restorative materials and graft versus host disease (Fig. 209).

*Diagnosis*

Incisional biopsy.

*Management*

Elimination of drugs, removal of restorative materials, further treatment for graft versus host disease (GVHD).

## Orofacial granulomatosis

*Aetiology and pathology*

May be a specific disease entity or may be associated with Crohn's disease. Non-caseating granulomas are seen on oral biopsy. Allergy to food constituents such as benzoates and cinnamaldehyde is common.

*Diagnosis*

Lip swelling (Fig. 210), angular cheilitis, full-width gingivitis, mucosal tags and irregular ulcers. Histological presence of granulomas.

*Management*

Exclusion diet, systemic or intralesional steroids.

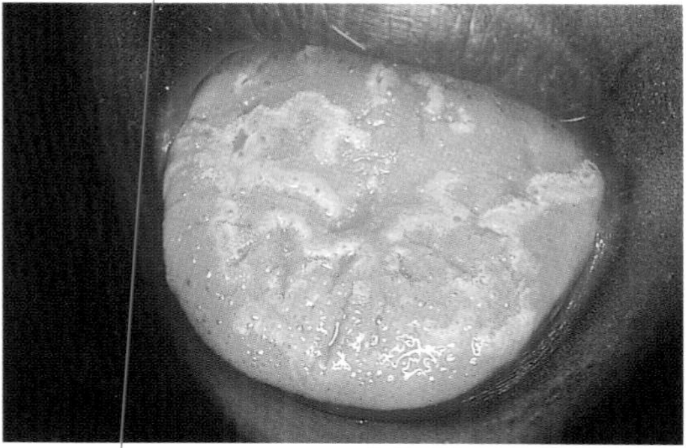

**Fig. 208** Geographic tongue.

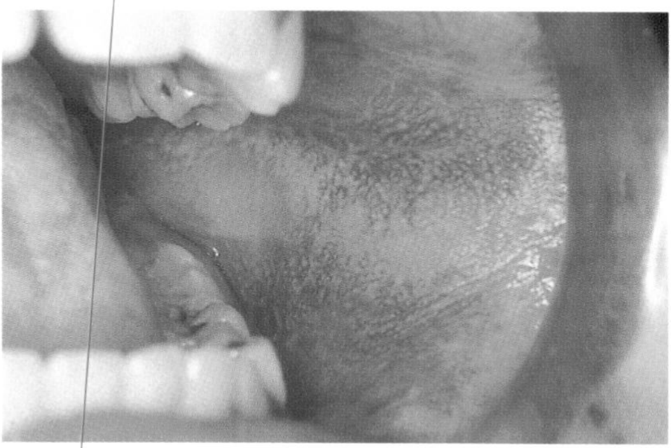

**Fig. 209** Lichen planus.

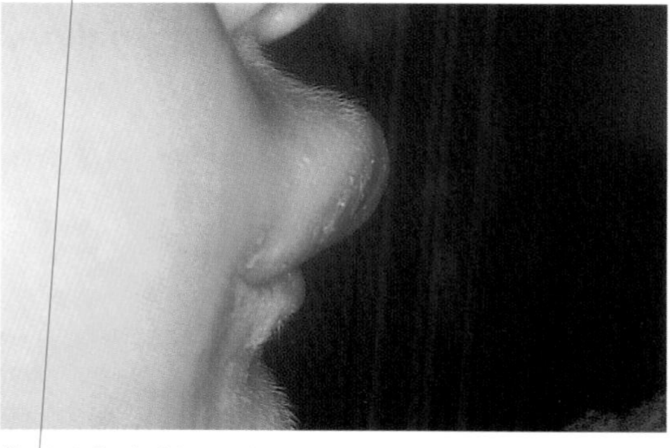

**Fig. 210** Orofacial granulomatosis with upper lip swelling.

## Pericoronitis

*Aetiology and pathology*

Inflammation of the operculum over an erupting tooth.

Associated trauma from a tooth in the opposing arch is usually present.

*Diagnosis*

Pain, trismus, swelling and halitosis. The operculum is swollen, red and often ulcerated 211). Fever and regional lymphadenitis may be present.

*Management*

Grinding or extracting opposing tooth and the local application of caustic agents (trichloracetic acid and glycerine).

Systemic antibiotics may be required.

## Denture stomatitis

*Aetiology and pathology*

Poor appliance hygiene, trauma from an ill-fitting appliance and *Candida albicans*.

*Diagnosis*

Diffuse erythema associated with the appliance base, often asymptomatic (Fig. 212).

*Management*

- Correct oral and appliance hygiene and adjust ill-fitting appliances.
- Soak the appliance overnight in hypochlorite solution.
- Use of antifungals such as amphotericin, miconazole and nystatin.

## Infective papilloma

*Aetiology and pathology*

Human papilloma virus (HPV).

*Diagnosis*

Papillomatous cauliflower-like appearance (Fig. 213). Common on palate, gingiva and oral mucosa.

*Management*

Spontaneous regression or excision.

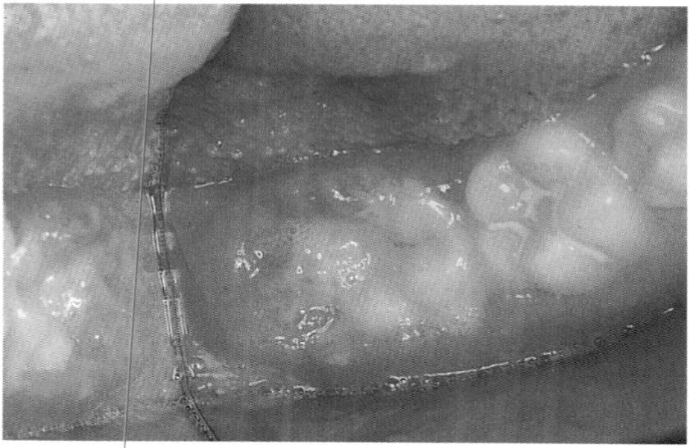

Fig. 211 Pericoronitis.

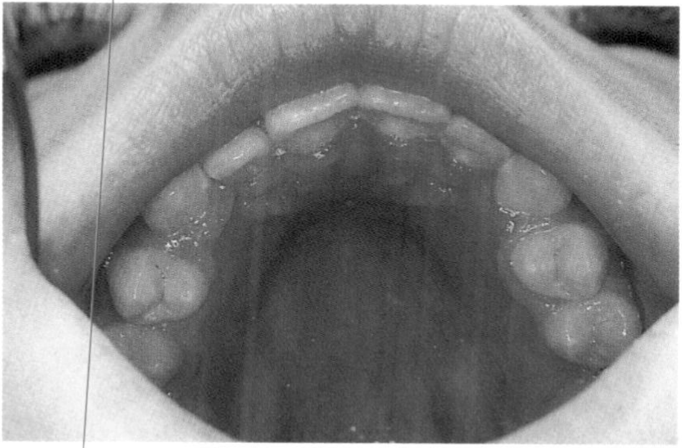

Fig. 212 Denture stomatitis.

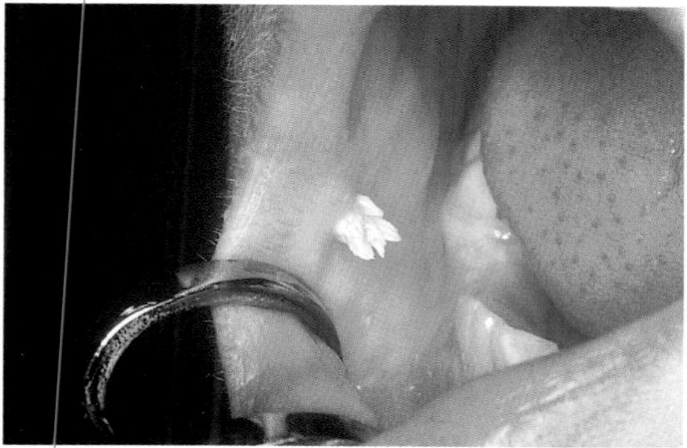

Fig. 213 Infective papilloma.

## Periapical infection

*Aetiology and pathology*

An abscess is often a sequel of pulpitis caused by dental caries or trauma. Mixed bacterial flora.

*Diagnosis*

Pain and facial swelling is characteristic (Fig. 214).

Intraoral swelling is common on the labial or buccal gingiva adjacent to the non-vital tooth (Figs 215, 216), but may occur on the palate in relation to the upper lateral incisors and the palatal root of the first permanent molars.

Occasionally abscesses of the lower incisors or molars may discharge extraorally.

*Management*

Extraction or endodontic therapy of the affected tooth.

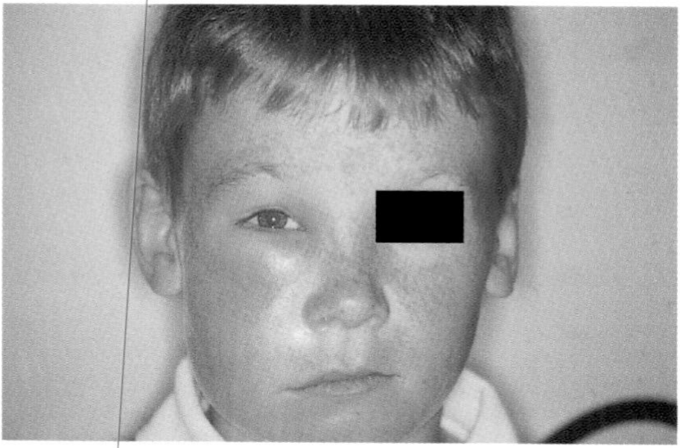

Fig. 214 Facial swelling resulting from periapical infection of a permanent incisor.

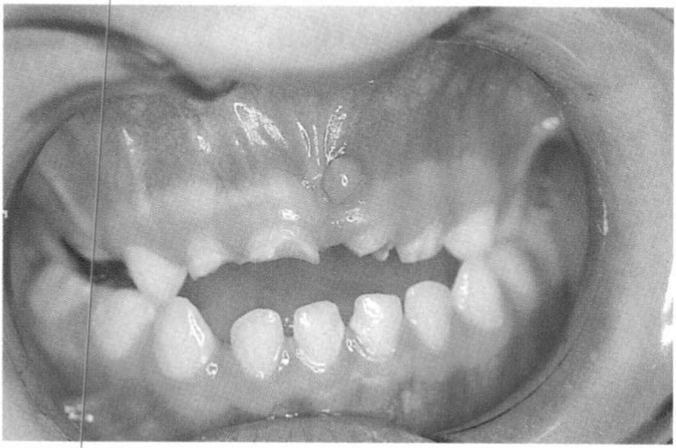

Fig. 215 Periapical infection of a primary incisor.

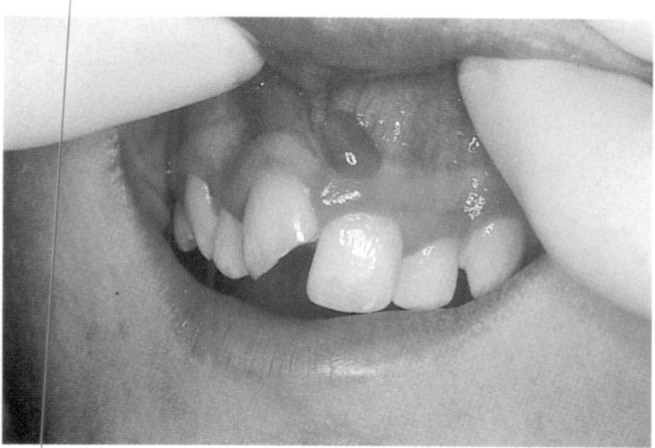

Fig. 216 Periapical infection of a permanent incisor.

# Recommended reading

## Orthodontics

Mitchell L 1996 An introduction to orthodontics. Oxford University Press, Oxford

Houston WJB, Stephens CD, Tulley WJ 1992 A textbook of orthodontics, 2nd edn. Wright, Oxford

Jones ML, Oliver RG 1997 Walther and Houston's orthodontic notes, 5th edn. Wright, Oxford

Shaw WC 1993 Orthodontics and occlusal management. Butterworth-Heinemann, Oxford

McDonald F, Ireland AJ 1998 Diagnosis of the orthodontic patient. Oxford University Press, Oxford

Proffit WR 1999 Contemporary orthodontics. Mosby Year Book Inc., St Louis

## Paediatric Dentistry

Scully C, Welbury RR 1994 A colour atlas of oral disease in children and adolescents. Wolfe Publications, London

Welbury RR ed. 1997 Paediatric dentistry. Oxford University Press, Oxford

Andreasen JO, Andreasen FM 1994 Textbook and colour atlas of traumatic injuries of the teeth, 3rd edn. Munksgaard, Copenhagen

# Index